Aidan Macfarlane is Director of the National Adolescent and Student Health Unit based in Oxford, and a Consultant in Public Health Medicine. His other books include *The Psychology of Childbirth* and *A Pocket Consultant in Child Health*.

Ann McPherson is a General Practitioner with extensive experience in advising students through her Oxford practice. Her other books include *Women's Problems in General Practice* and *Miscarriage* (with Ann Oakley and Helen Roberts).

They are together the authors of *Mum, I Feel Funny, Me and My Mates, The Virgin Now Boarding*, and the runaway bestsellers *The Diary of a Teenage Health Freak*, and *I'm a Health Freak Too!*

Steven Appleby's cartoons appear regularly in the *Guardian*, the *Oldie*, and the *Saturday Times Review*. His other books include *Rockets: A Way of Life by Captain J. Star, 99 Don'ts: A Guide to Unrecommendable Practices, 122 Turn Offs*, and *Normal Sex*.

GW00727880

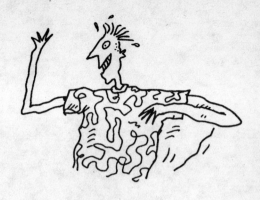

YOU'RE WONDERFUL

YOU'RE FANTASTIC

YOU'RE THE GREATEST

YOU'VE MADE IT

YOU'RE ON THE WAY TO THE TOP

YOU'RE OUT OF THIS WORLD

YOUR PARENTS THINK YOU'RE ACE

YOUR FRIENDS ARE ALL ENVIOUS

YOUR TEACHERS ARE ASTOUNDED

YOU'RE UP AND RUNNING

IN FACT YOU'RE THE BEST

OK—BUT . . .

HOW
ARE YOU
GOING TO
COPE AT
COLLEGE AND
SURVIVE
THE . . .

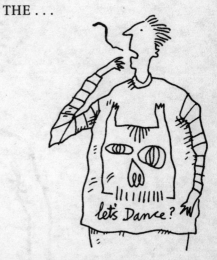

let's Dance?

*f*resher

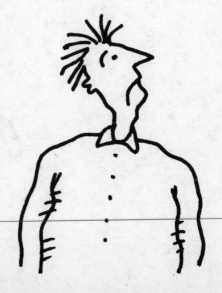

Pressure

How to survive as a
student

Aidan Macfarlane and Ann McPherson

OXFORD UNIVERSITY PRESS
1994

Oxford University Press, Walton Street, Oxford OX2 6DP

Oxford New York
Athens Auckland Bangkok Bombay
Calcutta Cape Town Dar es Salaam Delhi
Florence Hong Kong Istanbul Karachi
Kuala Lumpur Madras Madrid Melbourne
Mexico City Nairobi Paris Singapore
Taipei Tokyo Toronto

and associated companies in
Berlin Ibadan

Oxford is a trade mark of Oxford University Press

Text © Aidan Macfarlane and Ann McPherson 1994
Illustrations © Steven Appleby 1994

First published 1994 as an Oxford University Press paperback

All rights reserved. No part of this publication may be reproduced,
stored in a retrieval system, or transmitted, in any form or by any means,
without the prior permission in writing of Oxford University Press.
Within the UK, exceptions are allowed in respect of any fair dealing for the
purpose of research or private study, or criticism or review, as permitted
under the Copyright, Designs and Patents Act, 1988, or in the case of
reprographic reproduction in accordance with the terms of the licences
issued by the Copyright Licensing Agency. Enquiries concerning
reproduction outside these terms and in other countries should be
sent to the Rights Department, Oxford University Press,
at the address above

This book is sold subject to the condition that it shall not, by way
of trade or otherwise, be lent, re-sold, hired out or otherwise circulated
without the publisher's prior consent in any form of binding or cover
other than that in which it is published and without a similar condition
including this condition being imposed on the subsequent purchaser

British Library Cataloguing in Publication Data
Data available

Library of Congress Cataloging in Publication Data
Data available
ISBN 0–19–286167–0

10 9 8 7 6 5 4 3 2 1

Printed in Great Britain by
Clays Ltd.
Bungay, Suffolk

Very many thanks to . . .

. . . the hundreds of students who answered our advertisements, particularly — Rachel Coulter, Olly Minton, Harriet Sansom, Katherine Tulloh, Jojo Tulloh , Kirstin Ahmed, Hugo Thurston, Clare Sheehy, Jennifer Bobrow, and Jemma Blair; and all the McPherson and Macfarlane children, Beth, Tamara, Tess, Sam, Magnus, and Gus — for their special input.

And also to . . .

. . . Chris Bulstrode for his help with 'sports injuries', Keith Hawton for his help with 'suicide', Mary Marzillier for her help with 'work organization', Ken Wood for his help with 'exercise', Danby Bloch for his help with 'money', Deborah Waller and Chris Fairburn for their help with 'eating disorders', Phil Robson for his help with 'drugs', Nicky Lacey for her help with 'harassment', Jane Brown for the diet questionnaire, the Keith Durrant Project For Cancer Prevention for information on smoking, Ann Oakley and Gillian Bendelow for information on 'what worries teenagers', Fiona Palmer, Julia Allen, Ros Dunkley, Sue Weston, Adele Wright, Amanda Johnstone, Sally Crowe, Sharon Withnell, and Rachel Day for research and help (both wittingly and unwittingly), Sir David Weatherall for continuing to believe that we know what we are talking about, and Klim McPherson for still being there despite it all.

And to . . .

. . . Marny Leech for her everlasting patience and humour in editing and making general observations on life and the book, without making us feel too bad about our mistakes.

Sources . . .

Health Education Authority leaflets including: 'Enjoy Healthy Eating', 'Vaginal Infections', 'Minor Illness: How To Treat It At Home', 'That's the Limit', 'Herpes', 'Gonorrhoea', 'Genital Warts', 'Chlamydia', 'NSU', 'Thrush', 'Cystitis', 'AIDS Dialogue'; their books on adolescent health including *Today's Young Adults*; pamphlets from the Terrence Higgins Trust; Family Planning Association leaflets including: 'Your Choices — Contraception'; *The Pill* by John Guillebaud (Oxford University Press);

Sexual Health In Britain by Kaye Wellings *et al.* (Penguin); 'Managing Anxiety', a booklet by Gillian Butler; 'Coping With Anxiety: a Guide to Cognitive Therapy', a manual by Helen Kennerly; *Bulimia Nervosa* by Peter J. Cooper (Robinson Health); *Forbidden Drugs* by Phil Robson (Oxford University Press); National Union of Student publication, 'Coping With Abortion'; BPAS leaflet on 'Abortion'; Royal College of Psychiatrists leaflet 'Managing Anxiety and Phobias'; Oxford University Counselling Service handouts on 'Academic Work, Revision and Examinations'; *Eating Disorders: the Facts* by Suzanne Abraham and Derek Llewellyn Jones (Oxford University Press); 'Healthy Eating For Vegetarians' from the Oxfordshire Health Authority Nutrition and Dietetic Department; leaflets from the Institute For the Study Of Drug Dependence; 'Exercise, Why Bother?' from the HEA and Sports Council; 'Student Grants and Loans: a Brief Guide for Higher Education Students 1994/95' from the Department for Education; the *Oxford Textbook of Medicine* (Oxford University Press); and all the many other books, articles, magazines, papers where our filing system has failed us and we have not been able to make specific acknowledgements.

Wendy Cope's poem 'Some People' from *Making Cocoa for Kingsley Amis* is reproduced by kind permission of Faber and Faber Ltd.

Note

This book is for all students and 'would be' students at all types of college. It is a book in which much of the material has been written by students for students and put together with comments and information by the authors.

The quotes from students are all real, though sometimes the names have been changed and sometimes we have left the quotes anonymous. They were collected by a wide variety of means:

we put advertisements into student newspapers around the country and received a huge mailbag from which we chose what best represented the hopes, aspirations, and anxieties of students

we interviewed students just before they went up to university and when they came down at the end of their first term

we asked students to dictate 'diaries' for us onto tape machines during their Freshers' Week, to give us a minute-by-minute flavour of the action as it occurred, rather than seeing it through rose-tinted retrospective spectacles

we commissioned students to research specific topics

The material that we finally chose to go into the book was compiled from what we had learnt from direct face-to-face contact with students during our clinical work, from our research, from being parents of students, and from the huge correspondence we received.

Before completing the book, we asked a series of students — those about to go to university, those in their first year, and those finishing, to give an honest appraisal of the draft version — which they did!

Obviously we have not been able to cover every problem that every individual student might be faced with, but rather have tried to deal with the more common and practical aspects of college life. From our research with students it was clear that all students wanted to be considered as a student first, and a person with any type of 'problem' second. There are already extremely good sources of information for 'special interest groups' many of which are referred to in National Union of Students publications.

We hope you enjoy the results and that it relieves anxieties, confirms expectations, and entertains.

1

Anticipations, Expectations, and Worries

What are the anticipations and expectations?; things I'll miss; things I won't miss; advanced worries; enlarged worries; some other niggles; things to leave behind

2

Fresher Pressure

Famous parting shots; arrival; things you want to leave behind but will have difficulty managing; the first hours; the first week; going into action; things not to be seen with; the first term; if you feel like running away

3

Where to live, Where to hang out

Where to live; advanced tactics; what people say who have been through it already; sharing a telephone; preventing theft; where to hang out

4

Money

The hard graft of it; necessary action; the experiences of others; how students cope with money; grants; money tips for new students; budgeting

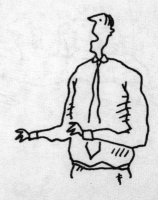

5

Friends

What students say about: making your first friends; the ethnic question; a sense of isolation; romantic involvements; different types at university; friends left behind

6

Sex and Relationships

A lecture note on sex; students' experiences of: sexual advances; straight and gay sex; shyness; celibacy

7

What degree would you get in contraception?

Test your knowledge on sex and contraception

8

'I promise I won't come . . .'

A 'quickie's guide' to the choices of contraception; emergency contraception; condoms; supercharging your sex life; the pill; the cap; other methods; 'I'm late . . .'; all about abortion

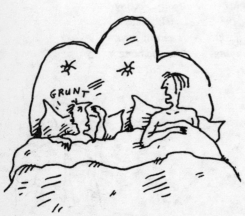

9

Food

Are you a nutritional disaster?; students' eating experiences; facts about fat, proteins and carbohydrates; vegetarian eating; cooking tips; a few easy recipes

10

Exercise and Sport

What physical fitness research shows; check your stamina; what various types of exercise are good for; aerobic and anaerobic sports; getting fit; overdoing it; sports injuries; uses and abuses of physiotherapy

11

Blowing your mind?

On drugs illegal; no need for speed; the need for speed; so how much do you know about drugs?; the facts and artefacts on all the commonly available drugs; overall damage limitation

12

Stress and Anxiety

What makes students stressed and anxious?; the results of stress and anxiety; managing anxiety; controlling a panic attack; overcoming worrying thoughts; coping with insomnia

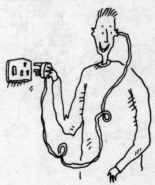

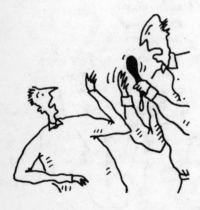

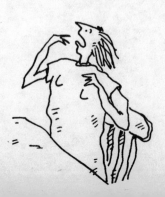

BEFORE ~

Why on earth
did I decide
to be a
student?

CHAPTER 1

Anticipations Expectations &worries

6 So many people and sources give the idea that university is about getting pissed every night, getting doped up to the eyeballs and rolling in and out of bed with anyone you possibly can.

Instead university is made up of a wide range of people, from different backgrounds, cultures and countries, all with different opinions and different reasons for being there. 9

6 The things I'm looking forward to most are also

What are the anticipations & expectations?

the things I worry about most — like I'm looking forward to meeting new people, but at the same time I don't want to meet new people. I like having friends but I don't like the effort of going into new rooms and meeting new people all the time. If I'm going to suss out who I'm going to get along with, I'll have to sift through a lot of strangers. I want to meet really nice, interesting people from different backgrounds but not go through the procedures.

'I can't wait for Freshers' Week — lots of parties and balls, very little sleep, spending money I haven't got, lots of drinking, looking around, with people willing to talk to anyone.'

Managing my own money will be a problem. Up till now, I've had pocket money weekly, but clothes and stuff basically my parents have paid for. Now it'll all be my own decisions — what I want to buy, when I want to buy it. I've saved some money from my holiday job, but I don't know what I'll spend it on yet.

Perhaps all I really want is just a few soulmates and not to be swamped by acquaintances. 〞

❝ I'm looking forward to freedom from my parents, and escaping from my home town. I want to be able to live away from home, with responsibility for my own finances and welfare. I can't wait to have a really good time without my mum and dad staying up until I get in.

I'm worried about making friends and managing my money, being thrown out of my digs, not being able to cook anything.

The essentials will be condoms, Tampax, and fags, an inflatable life-raft for emergencies, the *Radio Times*, photograph albums, and my *Beano* collection. **❯**

'I'll miss my mum and dad bailing me out (like when I lose my contact lenses), family life and home cooking.'

❛ I'm looking forward to interacting with new people and making a completely fresh start. Also to having a break from my teachers and parents, and having a room of my own which I can do anything in, at any time.

I worry about the workload, the pressures of exams and getting the work done on time, being alone, and getting lost — on or off campus.

Essential will be music and my teddy bears, especially my large ET who I can beat up at times of relative tension. Also essential are my frying pan and my own pillow. **〞**

❛ **I'm looking forward to more sex, more drink, a higher standard of sport,** meeting new people, getting away from crap teachers, playing for a good rugby team, and cheaper beer. AIDS is a worry and meeting dodgy people; also not being able to cope. I'll take with me toothpaste, food and money; and won't miss much from home. ❜

❛ **I'm not looking forward to going because of accounting for myself, being on my own and not sharing a room with my sister.** I think I will be very lonely. I want a direct phone link to my mum and dad. I'm also afraid of failing. I want a year's supply of clean underwear and teabags. Worries? The fact that everyone else will know what they're doing, and then money, money, money. ❜

❛ **I can't wait for the new social scene, getting into good sports because my school has lousy clubs, leaving my boring home town, trying cannabis.**

My list of worries? Not enough money, isolation, having to work harder than at school, meeting lots of weirdos, STDs, no holiday jobs, lousy accommodation, and exams. Also not being able to handle the pressure, not being the apple of my parents' eye, my sister getting one up on me.

After two years off working, just the idea of being able to wear tracksuit bottoms, trainers, and a T-shirt with "Pretentious – who – moi?" written across it. I can't wait to join the football team and the debating society, start a basketball team, take on the rest of the university, go underwater diving, do an aerobics class every day; have long, totally irrelevant, highly affected and supposedly philosophical arguments all night — and at last get away with acting like a student because I'll be one!

The terms are so short that you're on holiday most of the time — sounds good to me. Apart from having no money, the whole place sounds like heaven. People can stay whenever they want, the college looks beautiful, I'll be discovering a whole new city and meeting people from the four corners of the earth — all thrown together to get on or not, as we please.

It'll be interesting to see who got through at the interview, and who'll be in the room next door (I hope they have a TV). 9

Things I'll miss . . .

- friends
- my boyfriend/girlfriend
- my cat
- mum/dad
- my meals cooked for me
- phone calls for me
- using the family car
- my parents paying for things

Things I won't miss . . .

- loud parents
- being told what to do
- having to clear up the mess in my room (why do I have to clear up my room when the whole world's in a mess?)
- my parents wanting to know where I am
- nasty people who I've hated for years

Advanced worries

'You worry about insignificant things, like my favourite worry at the moment is where I'm going to get the key to my room. My ten best worries are: what am I going to do on my first night? Who do I try and talk to first? Money — and how I work out a budget. Will there be any other people like me there? How many people in my block will be in my year? Who will I get on with? How do I get money when my cheques run out? Do I turn up in my jeans? Do they expect me to know everything already? And where am I going to get my key?

It's all the practical things like that — nothing major, I know.'

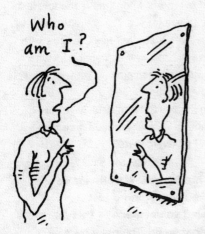

Enlarged worries

'No advance personal contact from anyone. It would have been nice if they'd sent somebody round, or phoned. I'd have appreciated that — especially if they'd said, "I know that it's going to be pretty daunting. Here you are, just sit down and I'll explain."

There was all this stuff from the Dean and the Finance Officers, people I've never met writing me little bureaucratic missives. I could see that at the top of all the letters they'd changed the date from "August 1993" to "August 1994". I know you need to get a certain amount of information across, but it could be done in a more friendly way.'

❝ I'm not worried about the work — just about silly things like what am I going to do on the first night? And how am I going to get to the university from where I am now? The second night there's a disco laid on, and on the third, a cheese and wine party organized by a bank. I think that's a good idea. It would also be nice to know that there was an unofficial gathering in someone's room. I won't know about that till I get down there.

Once you've got one person you're talking to, you're fine. If there's two of you, you can approach anyone you like! ❞

'The real stress is going there and looking like a headless chicken — totally lost. You wish there was someone there who'd tell you what to do and metaphorically hold your hand. It might be only the first two or three hours that you feel like this, but you probably can't expect to feel all right for two or three weeks. **When you've met up with one or two other people, it doesn't matter where you are or what you're doing.**'

'**I suppose money worries me a bit. I don't know which bank to sign up with** — it will depend on which one has a branch on the campus. The one I'm with at the moment has given me the usual bribes — £25 and a four hundred quid overdraft. I don't have the foggiest how to budget yet. I'm going to stay away from a student loan, to start with at least, but it will all depend on what my parents can come up with, won't it? At the moment I don't think I'll get into loans because I can usually get by without. I've always made sure that I never go overdrawn.'

'**About making friends — well, not so much making friends, more just getting to chat to someone — this is always hardest to do.** There's a huge barrier between you and the first person you come across. Once you're past that, you're up and running and nobody is going to knock you down. You just get in there, do everything, and enjoy yourself.'

6 **Fitting in may be a real problem. What shall I do if they are all rugger buggers in suits and I'm there in my tatty gear?** When I sort it all out in my mind, I realize they can't all be rugger buggers and won't all come in suits — after all, fifty per cent of them are going to be girls. One part of me knows that this is not worth worrying about, but then it creeps into my mind again and has to be dealt with. In fact, I'll probably walk in and there'll be a cross-section of everyone. I know that's what's going to happen really, but these other thoughts just keep coming into my head. **9**

6 **Will people like me? Most of my friends come from a similar background to me, and have been to state schools — but when I get to university, they'll have come from different backgrounds —** at least I hope they will. I hope there'll be a massive cross section — there's nothing worse than a narrow, middle-class outlook and an idealistic view of life. The sort of person I would like to meet is someone who has worked hard to get there, but I've promised to go in there with a completely open mind. **9**

Some other niggles

'I want to be sent a list of people sharing my flat with me so that I can contact them ahead of time.'

'Will I be completely brainwashed by university, change completely, and not realize it?'

'I worry about getting into situations with someone of the opposite sex and not being able to deal with them.'

'Did I make the right choice about my course, and will I be able to change it?'

Things to leave behind . . .

- your old boyfriend or girlfriend
- your inhibitions
- worries that everyone else knows what they are doing and you don't
- your brand new, super deluxe, 24-gear, hydroelastic suspension mountain bike
- your 'NOW' tapes

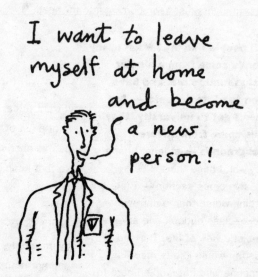

I want to leave myself at home and become a new person!

CHAPTER 2

FRESHER
PRESSURE

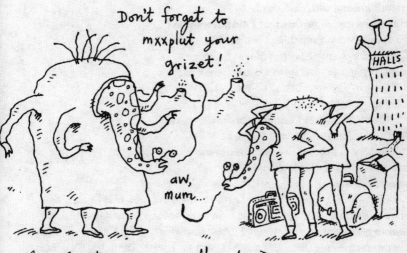

Don't forget to mxxplut your grizet!

aw, mum...

HALLS

Mrs Monster says goodbye to Doreen.

Famous parting shots . . .

Mum and Dad:

'We'll be back to see you soon.'

'If you can't be good, be careful.'

'Clean your teeth.'

'I don't know how we're going to cope without you.'

'Don't forget to eat.'

'Have you got enough clean underpants?'

'Did you remember to pack your . . .?'

'Phone us tonight and let us know how you are getting on.'

'Don't forget that we are proud of you.'

'Make sure that you get enough sleep.'

'Don't do anything I wouldn't do.'

Famous parting shots . . .

Students:

'OK, yup, umh, see ya!'

Arrival

'The last few days at home were a nightmare and with each day I convinced myself further that I did not want to go to university. Everything I had read about the first week or so there portrayed it as the worst week of your life — alone in a barren room, not speaking to anyone, missing home, and a catalogue of other horrors.

I can honestly say I cannot relate to this at all. My first week stands out as a highlight. Admittedly, at times I felt a bit insecure and lost, but otherwise I settled into student life with remarkable ease. I don't consider myself someone who finds it easy to make friends, yet this really wasn't a problem. My "corridor" mates were friendly and we all got on well instantly. Everyone else I met, in hall and on campus, was also friendly and talkative. After all, everyone wants to make friends, even if they don't always feel able to. Both the university and hall made it easy to mix, and there were lots of organized events. '

'When I arrived, the place was really quiet. As soon as I got to my room, I wanted Dad to leave. I wanted to get started and get out there, so when he'd gone I went for a walk over to the Students' Union. It was all locked up and there was no one there, so I came back feeling rather miserable. However, there was this note under my door which said, "Dear Fresher — thirsty, bored, sober? Come over to Room 413."

Well, I wasn't going to sit in my room all evening! Thinking I was bound to meet someone there, I walked across and came to this tiny room packed with people. You couldn't move. I walked in, someone stuck a bottle of wine into my hand, and I didn't look back.

When the wine had gone, it was straight down to the bar. It turned out they were all fresher dentists. The next day there was a party at the Union, the day after one at my department, the day after that another party at the Union. There were no bad times at all! '

❝ **I arrived at university with my new teapot, the relevant bits of paper, some "year off" stories, a healthy suntan, and the enthusiasm to get into it all and make a massive number of really great friends.** Unfortunately, this is not as easy as you might think and, for me, Freshers' Week turned into a nightmare.

There was continual consumption of free alcohol and coffee, and everyone was either desperately over-friendly or aloof. I didn't feel I was communicating with anyone, and my year off caught up with me in the form of dysentery.

I was continually half-drunk and buzzing on caffeine; also making endless trips to the toilet and daily journeys to the doctor with stool samples for testing. On top of all this, there were so many things to organize. I kept missing vital "signing in" sessions and was constantly in the wrong place at the wrong time.

I don't think I've ever felt so close to becoming insane as I did during that first mad week. The main feeling was of loneliness and the strain of keeping a constant grin on my face when I felt completely distraught.

I later found out that although there were some people like me (pretending to enjoy it all and feeling that the moment you admitted that everything was not simply great, you had failed), the majority really were enjoying getting pissed, having inane conversations, and the boarding school/camp atmosphere of corridor parties in impersonal halls of residence.

These latter are now bored with university — whereas I am boundlessly happy, with some solid friendships. ❞

❝ **It wasn't easy, that's for sure.** Life was one mass of confusion from Day One. I was left rather tearfully by my long-term boyfriend amidst a litter of boxes and suitcases in an alien world — a block full of females who all seemed to be coping better than me. Don't get me wrong. I'm hardly innocent and not particularly family orientated, so I expected to be able to cope. But being a fresher is indeed a nightmare, in spite of all the efforts of the university authorities.

Freshers' Week passed with chasing round the campus after forms and signatures, and with introductory lectures. After the secure environment of home, it was all a bit bewildering, and during the first few days there were moments when I felt like packing it in and catching the next train home. Then came some real friends and now I wouldn't give it up for the world.

The first girl I met, who I thought would turn into a friend, I haven't seen for ages. As the desperation receded, I could start being myself again and stop putting on a front. People like to say they are having a wild time when, in many cases, if they are honest, they are insecure and petrified. The girls I was jealous of in Freshers' Week because I thought they were coping, are now afraid to go out and find new opportunities and are not being honest about their fears. **If we had talked about these fears together, we would all have got over them much more quickly.** 9

6 **The moment had arrived — it was a quarter past one in the afternoon. The trip down here was horrendous.** When it came to the point, I didn't want to go to university and when I had to pack all my stuff up I felt like I was leaving for ever and never coming back. I cried my eyes out all the way, but luckily we had my boyfriend Jim with us, and he looked after me.

I think the very worst bit of arriving was walking into my room. There was no heating, it was pouring with rain, and all I wanted to do was go home. I thought, "Oh no, this is my place for ever," and it's the ultimate downer when all that place has got is breeze-block walls, a bed, a table, and a wardrobe. It just looked awful.

Once I had got my stuff in, and my mother and Jim had left, I sorted it all out and it wasn't so bad. I tried not to think about the fact that they had gone. I put my pictures up and my bits and pieces all around and the room looked much better. Their leaving was terrible. I wanted them to go immediately because I can't handle long goodbyes. Jim was crying and I was crying. It was awful.

I was much happier when I had met some of the other girls. We immediately introduced ourselves and everyone was friendly. I had been so scared about what these girls were going to be like — normal or weird and into completely different things from me, but they were really great. There are eight of us in my flat, but one girl doesn't mix. We all went out to the bar in our hall. There were hordes of students there. It was unbelievable — it took us an hour to get a drink. We just chatted to all and sundry and everyone, well nearly everyone, was friendly. The blokes, who are all downstairs, are really nice but the girls across the corridor, who are in the year above, just don't want to know us. We have to answer the phone for them. I think that's completely off. 9

Things you may want to leave behind but will have difficulty managing . . .

♦ your parents making you feel guilty

♦ your acne

♦ your overdraft

♦ your shyness

♦ the look on your mother's face when she departs

❛ I've rung my mum. She can't believe I'm actually quite happy! I can't believe it myself — I thought I would be bound to be homesick. Mum's pretty upset, because she's now on her own and feels lonely. I'll miss Jim, and I've written to him already so that he doesn't feel left out.

The first hours . . .

My feelings at the moment are in complete and utter disarray. I've got to go bed now, in a strange bed in a strange room surrounded by people I don't really know. It's almost frightening! ❜

Remember:

▶ two jars of instant coffee — one for borrowing, one for yourself

▶ a packet of condoms (they come in three sizes — small, medium and liar)

▶ your bank account

▶ Mars bars for when trekking across vast empty spaces

▶ your self-confidence

. . . and the first week

Monday

'I seem to have spent most of today signing up for things in Freshers' Week, as well as getting my Union Card and looking around. All the paperwork is a bit boring but it has to be done. I talked to my mum again today and that was great. She's feeling better about me being here now, and I'm still happy!

I registered for my course today — more queueing. I met two girls who are also taking it (I jumped in with both feet and talked to them both as I didn't know anyone else on it) and two guys. They are definitely not my type. Most of the people on my course are 24 or over — and there are only six girls. This freaked me out as I was hoping to meet someone nice to go around with. When I got back to the flat, the others had all met really great people. The ones I'd met hadn't given me much more than the time of day.

I haven't joined any clubs yet as I don't know what interests me and I won't know anyone there. I guess that's the whole point — you go there to meet people! I don't know if I can do that yet. I'm a bit scared. My mum said that she feels like this even now.

It's great having someone I like next door because we look after each other. If I feel upset she comes in. The other girls are great too. We all go out together every evening until late. Everything's all going quite well.'

Tuesday

'I've just got in and I'm knackered with signing up for things again. I've signed up for basketball which should be fun, and a friend in the flat is going to do it with me. I got up this morning and didn't have anything to do till one o'clock. It was a depressing experience. Everyone else had gone out so I just sat in my room, feeling lonely. All my old friends were at work so I couldn't phone them. I wandered around thinking, "What am I doing here?"

I had a meeting of my course to go to later but I wasn't looking foward to that as I don't much like the other people on it. So I wrote some letters to friends to keep my mind off this and to stop me thinking.

In the evening we went to a Bavarian Night at the Union. It was absolutely ace with loads of people. I haven't had such a good time in ages. I spoke to my mum after supper. She's OK, but I miss her like crazy. We never used to get on, but ever since I've been here, we've got on brilliantly. **It's really weird. I don't know what it'll be like when I get home again.'**

Thursday

'Jim's written every day, telling me absolutely everything, which I love. I might get bored with it after a bit, though. Some of the things he's doing with our friends make me feel a bit left out, but I do have another life up here now.

I asked the others if they'd like to go into town with me, but they had scheduled things to do all day so there was me all by myself in the flat again. It was awful. Everyone else seems to have made lots of friends. Maybe it's just me. I don't seem to be doing as well as they are. I guess it will all come in time.

I talked to Jim on the phone

today. There was no one else in his house so
he rang me back. We talked for ages. I miss
him like crazy and bawled my eyes out. He's
got a week off soon and might come and see
me. Not sure this is a good idea. I'd be very
happy to see him, but when he goes away
again it might unsettle me. I feel reasonably
settled at the moment.'

Saturday

**'I got up really late. It's wonderful to have
the freedom to lie in bed without Mum
nagging.** No one got up till one o'clock. We all
went shopping in the afternoon. It was good fun
walking around, just exploring.

I do miss the food at home. The meals here
are not bad, but it's all such a hassle — set
times, and half the time you're not really
hungry. None of us are enjoying the food.

I miss the space at home too, and the
security. It's terrible getting back here at night.
People say you shouldn't walk, so I have to
take the bus and it's 80p. I'm going to have to
cut down on going out because of money.'

Going into action

➤ find a 'friend' — anyone will do, just an acquaintance, someone to
talk to, a bit of mutual consolation over the rigours of the first week. It
doesn't have to last

➤ get a phone card — that is, if your parents haven't thought about this
already. It is invaluable to be able to contact the outside world easily
at times of crisis (and even not at times of crisis)

➤ get a library card — student card, student rail card (in fact, any useful cards going). It looks great when you unreel them from your wallet, and they all come in useful at one time or another

➤ open a bank account — shop around. You're 90 per cent sure to need an overdraft (see Chapter 4), so find out who will give you the best deal. Don't be bribed by the odd shiny pencil or Smith's token. It may not feel like it, but in the long run they want your business. There are, after all, lots of banks to choose from

You need to decide on:

◗ who gives you the highest free overdraft?

◗ who charges the least bank charges?

◗ who has the most convenient branch for where you live?

◗ what are their 'hole in the wall' facilities like?

◗ do they treat you like a grown-up human being and show you the right degree of politeness?

➤ Find out where the local chemist and local shop are — especially those that are open outside normal hours. It is inevitable that you will run out of milk, sanitary towels, baked beans, instant coffee, and cornflakes (though with luck not usually all at the same time) at three o'clock in the morning.

➤ Register with a doctor — one you like and feel at ease with. Different universities have different arrangements with family doctors. Some have a central medical service with 'dedicated' doctors, some have arrangements with local GPs, some just leave it up to you. When you get to university, it is a good idea to register with a doctor (rather like opening a bank account for your health instead of money); even if you never need to see one, at least you will have a 'safety net'. Don't worry, however, if you don't register and you do need one. Doctors will always be available. If you don't like your college doctor, you are perfectly free to find some other GP you do like and feel you can talk to.

'The trip to the medical centre with all its past connotations of fierce nit inspectors and immunization needles loomed large in my list of fears.** One of those Hieronymus Bosch images that will remain with me for the rest of my life was the sight of hundreds of white-faced freshers trying to hold pretentious conversations and water samples simultaneously in the medical queue and still retain their street credibility.'

'I registered with a local GP — a brilliant move as it was good to have a sympathetic ear** outside the bureaucratic environment of the campus, and away from the world that often in itself creates a sense of ill-being. However, after talking to my friends later, it turned out that the student health centre was just what they wanted — so be sure to choose what suits you.'

'The great advantage of the university doctor** was that she deals with students all the time. She was great at talking to my tutor when I hadn't done some work because I'd been ill. She knew just how to handle it.'

Things not to be seen with . . .

- your teddy bear
  - a copy of the *Financial Times*
    - a mug with John Major on it
      - a potty with a picture of the queen

❝ **They actually did come knocking on your door to make sure you didn't just stew away in your** **. . . and finally the first term** **own loneliness** — but they didn't force you at all. Most of the people I got to know weren't living in the same block as me, which worried me at first; but now I'm reaping the advantages because I can get a bit of peace and quiet when I want it.

Where we're living is not the most architecturally pleasing building I've ever seen. Basically, I use where I live just to sleep. The hospital canteen is surprisingly good and cheap, so I only cook myself when I've got friends over.

Books are pricey. I bought the basics but use the library for the rest. They're great at the library. They explain where everything is and how to use it, and they're really friendly. It's awful the way that some of the books there just seem to disappear. We are frisked when we leave and I've heard that at some universities they won't give you your degree until you've returned all your library books!

Some people have found it difficult — the shock of it all, being thrown in at the deep end and being confronted by a load of drunken slobs. A standard initiation is "ginning": eight singles in a glass, down in one, stand the person on a chair, rotate them and leave. This is considered "entertainment"! **9**

6 Coming back home at the end of the first term, it was like half of me had never been away. The first thing I did was pick up the phone to my friends, and then it was, "See you down the pub in twenty minutes." It got to eleven o'clock when the pubs close and everything went dead. Not like London! This was outrageous. I can't go to sleep at eleven o'clock. At college, an early night is 1 a.m., a late night, 4 a.m. I'm just about living on no sleep, and I was on "college time" when I got home. Gradually I got back to normal, but I can't wait to get back there. **9**

6 I've got four tutors for each subject and I see each of them with twelve other students. I have an academic tutor too, and a personal tutor, in case I have any problems.** Everyone is encouraged to make contact with their personal tutor. Also on site is a counselling service and an occupational health service. I've met all these people and they seem a very friendly bunch.

To begin with, I had a substitute mum as well (a second-year student) which was rather a bizarre experience. At first I couldn't find her as I didn't know who she was, then she suddenly came up to me and said, "I'm your mum, come and have a cup of tea." She told me all the things I had to do initially, but I haven't seen her since. The second-years were trying to be helpful, but it was early days to know what our problems were likely to be, and we hadn't started any proper work. **9**

6 Half of me would like to get to know everyone, but you can't and have to make do with a few. For instance, you meet someone you think you might really like and then you never see them again. In London, it's best to be on a campus near the centre, so that everything is five minutes walk down the road and you can use all these really cheap deals — like at the theatre. There are things going on on the campus as well — a bop every Friday and the bar is always open. You can become incredibly insular though if you just stay on campus. You need a life outside. **)**

'I feel much more appreciated than I did at school. There is something very "normal" about everything here. Before I came up, I was worried because a lot of the people who talked about university, talked about things I wasn't interested in, like drugs, sex, being cool. But it hasn't turned out to be like that.

I was also worried because I never liked going out in the sixth form. I found the whole social scene terrifying and thought university would be the same. But it isn't, and I enjoy the social side. **)**

And if you feel like running away . . .

- remember it will get better
- stick it out if you possibly can
- don't feel that you've got to expose yourself to the outside world of university all the time
- go for a walk, read a book, listen to your favourite music, take some exercise (see Chapter 10)
- remember lots of other people will be feeling the same way
- don't give up too soon
- ring your parents and friends from home
- get m to come and visit you at weekends
- talk to your tutors
- go and see the counselling services or your doctor

Postscript for staff

'*"We welcome you to this college with open arms", the Master says. "We want you to enjoy yourselves here, and get as much value out of university life as possible."*

I'm listening with rapt attention to the introductory speech in Freshers' Week, Intro Week — call it what you will. And, of course, I'm eager to make friends with everybody around me, and the Master seems like a good bloke.

"Look upon me as a friend. We are a friendly college and I am always willing to spend time with undergraduates if they should have any problems, or even if they just want a chat."

I took this advice to heart. The next day, while walking down the street, I saw the Master. "Hello", I said, in a friendly manner; **at which point he quickly looked away and continued to walk down the street.')**

where to LIVE
WHERE TO
HANG OUT

Where to live

Accommodation is very variable from university to university, and universities also differ over how many students get places in halls of residence for the first year.

It is worth putting a bit of effort into seeing whether you can find somewhere decent to live (in or out of hall). It will not only be your single most expensive item, but it will also be where you spend a considerable amount of your time.

Advance tactics

- find a friend, or a friend of a friend — someone who has been through it all at the same university — and ask advice

- ring the university accommodation office and ask for information

- fill in the forms that the university sends you about accommodation and return them as quickly as possible

- go and 'case' the halls when you visit, ask people in the corridors for advice — get the 'inside' story

- the best prepared will investigate accommodation as soon as they've got their results
- look in local newspapers for rented accommodation if you are going to live out
- read contracts on rented accommodation with care
- take advice over how much you can reasonably be expected to put down as a deposit

What people say who have been through it already

‘One of the good things about living in a hall of residence is that there is no need to buy your own hi-fi system. You can listen to the music that someone two rooms down the corridor or four floors up is playing.

In college there is no such thing as silence. Well, if you're lucky,

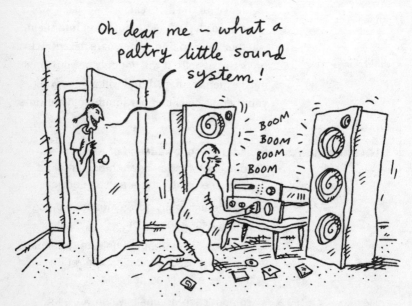

Oh dear me – what a paltry little sound system!

BOOM
BOOM
BOOM
BOOM

Meeting your neighbour in the hall of residence.

there might be a few minutes between 4.30 and 5.30 a.m. But outside those blissful moments, it is pointless trying to tell your neighbour to turn his music down because there's always someone else making just as much noise somewhere else in the building. And that twat is always playing Status Quo.

Once I can see there is no escape, I turn up the volume of my own hi-fi set. If I have to live and work in my room, I will do it to the sound of my own noise. Of course, nobody comes round to ask me to turn the music down. People either can't hear it, or I can't hear them knocking on the door. I have become part of the problem. **'**

LODGINGS Lonely, boring, difficult to meet other students, but good for independence once you know who you want to share with.

HALLS Halls are great. It's very easy to meet other students as everybody is so desperate to make friends. Events are organized so that students get the chance to interact.

LARGE HALLS have better and more facilities.

SMALL HALLS have a better community feel and are more homely.

WHERE TO LIVE

SELF-CATERING HALLS Nice because you can eat when, where and how you want. It's more expensive to buy food, though, than you might think. It also takes time to prepare meals, but at least this gets you away from doing work all the time. Good if you can get a cooking rota going between friends because you have much less hassle and you don't starve.

CATERED HALLS Nice because you don't have to bother about cooking food, or worry when you're going to get your next meal. But pain in the arse because meals are served at certain times and you have to arrange your life around them. The food can also be disgusting.

❛Our hall is split into flats with seven people in each. We share two toilets, a shower and a kitchen. This is nice because it feels like a little house and forces me to get to know people. It's quite amusing in my case because there's conflict between some of our flatmates at the moment, caused by the state of the kitchen and people using one another's plates, pots, and pans. **One girl has locked all her cutlery in her trunk!**❜

❛**I was one of the unfortunate few who was allocated a double room.** Initially I was excited at the prospect of sharing a room with somebody who was bound to be a kindred spirit, but I was sorely disappointed. Some bastard in the administration office obviously had an extremely malicious streak and must have thought it the height of amusement to put two people who are as different as chalk and cheese in a room together. It wasn't amusing to us. For someone who is essentially a night owl and doesn't surface until midday, it is not exactly conducive to friendship to be woken up at 6 a.m. each morning by the sound of his partner's alarm clock. Fortunately, after a term of living hell, I managed to wheedle myself into a single room!❜

❛**It was my first time away from home** and owing to a shortage of student accommodation I was allocated a room in a hotel, which I shared with another girl. At first this was excellent. I didn't know anybody in Bournemouth and I had just left a secure family life. The other girl was in the same boat. We became rather close friends, did everything together, and sat talking till late at night.❜

❛**I'm now living with three close friends in a nice, but cold, house. The living room is a serious exercise in bad taste. Maroon sofa (cushions attached with velcro), beige wallpaper (peeling rather than appealing), a chair that looks as though several B52s had used it for bombing practice,** and a big green cushion affectionately known as "hulk". We overcome these small adversities through humour — and through most of us being short-sighted! Ironically, our first caller was a market researcher doing a survey on furniture! At that point, we weren't up to suggesting that we'd done the interior from Harrods. **❜**

❛My first impression of my room was hysterical. I couldn't believe I'd been put there. It looked like a prison cell — just one narrow window with a ledge, a few box items supposed to be cupboards, and that was it. I nearly burst into tears. But I've grown to love it and now it's cosy and special.

Eight people in my flat share a very small kitchen and two loos. It's not much, but it really has become home and we all get on well. Posters are up on the wall (even if Blu-tack has been banned) and a phallic cactus called "Robert's Thing" is established near a window.

It's a big gamble. You could be made to live with people you don't get on with at all. And in a flat you have to make decisions together (about the TV, sharing the phone, cooking, washing-up). You also can't go locking up your cooking utensils and insisting you're the only one who can use them. Perhaps the most glaring problem that arises when sharing with seven other completely different people is the conflict between the "neaties" and the "messies". Some people like the flat to be spick and span, others like it messy because it feels homely — and they don't like to be told to clear their stuff up as they want complete freedom from "parents". Me? I'm in betweenish. I prefer it clean but can tolerate quite a bit of mess without becoming hysterical. It's hard to get a balance without some arguments. **❜**

❛Accommodation is perhaps the biggest hurdle of a fresher's year. It is an area where losers outnumber winners 6 to 1. The only really basic qualification that is useful is "spawniness" — that is, being able to fall into a cesspit and still come up smelling of roses.

Mine is a "federal" university where a student has two of everything including two accommodation officers. "Ah ha!", thinks the first-year innocent, "double the chances of finding a place of my own." Little do they know, as they saunter down to their local office, to be told, "Well, it's not really us you want, it's up to the central office." A sweaty journey to the central office — only to hear the magic words, "Deal with your local office first, and if you've no success, come back to us."

All this aside, one does occasionally find a gem. Even then there are problems, for here one is in May looking for places for September. Most landlords require a hefty deposit and for you to pay throughout the summer. Naturally, few students have the resources to pay rent for a place in which they will not be living. The best bet is to offer to pay a retainer in return for which the landlord will hold the property till September, but for heaven's sake get it in writing.

Flat hunting is a hassle. It seems that you have only just settled into your first-year accommodation and here you are having to find a new abode. Also, most students have to look for a new place while sitting their end-of-year exams, so a bottle of valium is an essential in any student flat hunter's rucksack. Be prepared to meet the kind of unscrupulous shark whom you have only ever seen profiled on Esther Rantzen's *That's Life.*

My first impressions were of long labyrinthine corridors with bathrooms, kitchens, bedrooms. It felt more like a hospital or an old people's home, **and it took a lot of courage to knock on my neighbour's door.** My friend was in a shared flat where everyone mucked in together. However, the advantage of my set-up was that I had more privacy.

Telephones are a **nightmare:**

- if you are sharing a phone, it always, always, always causes problems

- if you are sharing a phone which is not a pay phone, organize this before you move in. Write down what the arrangement is and get everyone to sign it. Make sure it is absolutely specific so that no one can claim they didn't understand at the beginning

- never be the person with ultimate responsibility for any contract. You inevitably get caught as the person who finally has to pay it for everyone else

SHARING A TELEPHONE:

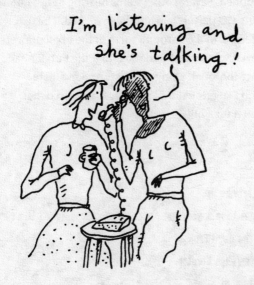

I'm listening and she's talking!

How to get around these problems:

- have a phone with incoming calls only (and make outgoing ones from a local phonebox)

- each have your own BT chargecard

- tell your parents you will phone home if they will give you a phonecard

- get an itemized phone bill

Theft can be a problem

' One Friday evening we had set the video to record *Whose Life Is It Anyway?* and had gone to the pub. When we staggered back in the early hours, the flat looked a complete mess as usual, but the video was nowhere to be seen. In our inebriated state, realization was slow to dawn that it had in fact been nicked. Eventually the penny dropped and the police were summoned. Several other items bearing plugs, notably a ghetto blaster and the CD player, had also been filched. The two constables took the details, looked around them at the open drawers with clothes strewn everywhere, and remarked that the burglar had given the place a pretty thorough going-over. Me and my mate exchanged glances and I suggested that actually it appeared that, if anything, they'd tidied it up a bit! **'**

How to prevent theft

■ **Lock everything up.**
The day you forget to lock your
door, will be the day that
Mr/Mrs/Ms/Master/Miss Burglar
decides to visit.

■ **Get insured** — if possible, under your
parents' home insurance policies (check this out with them).
Otherwise, there are companies which specialize in student
insurance and offer reasonable deals. You may not think you have
anything worth stealing, but add up the value of everything
you own, estimate how much it would cost to replace
it, and you may change your mind.

Where to hang out There will be moments when you want to be by yourself and other moments (for some, all of the time) when you want to snatch a 'gargleblaster' and exchange juicy notes with your mates.

❬ Let's say that I have actually done a piece of work and am feeling thoroughly satisfied with myself — then I'd probably head down to one of the campus bars, as they are always packed with atmospherics. There are one or two others that are smaller and more mellow, and do some damn fine cocktails. Then there's this other one full of sporty people, rugger buggers in suits playing drinking games, but I've only been there a couple of times. There's a nightclub on campus as well, called "The Hothouse", which is a bit of a gamble. It can be brilliant (on "70s Nights") or dire (on nights when they have to pump out the dry ice to hide the fact that hardly anyone is dancing).

Personally, I stick to the bars with atmospherics, such as the one with a pool table. I'm desperately trying to improve my skills, but I'm sick and tired of blokes (who've been playing since they were in nappies) telling me how I should be doing it. Occasionally me and my flatmates pop into town to see a film or take in a nightclub. I don't really know where the key places to be seen are. Maybe I'm not in with the trendy set, but I can live with that. ❭

❬ Most weekday evenings I go to my hall bar. I like it there because that's where all the people living near me hang out and I'm guaranteed to see someone I know well. The drinks are cheap which is good. I don't go out to get wasted. I just like having a drink and a chat with friends, and getting away from work for a while.

I do various things at weekends, like a couple of pubs, and very occasionally a club. I also like going out for meals, to the cinema, and to hear the odd band at a local venue. You don't necessarily have to make the big city at night, as campus offers most things. Often I don't even feel like going out, in which case I go and chat in someone's room,

putting down tons of biscuits and endless
cups of coffee made with the obligatory
Marvel milk. 9

▶ *Each others' rooms* — the best place for
slagging people off in a cosy intimate
atmosphere where you can really get down to
the nitty gritty. This needs to be with good
friends, and is obviously not the place to
meet new people outside your immediate
circle, but it is a good preparation before
going to face the outside world. Given the
size of most college rooms, if you are more
than four people, this may be very intimate.

**However, you may want to defend your room
from invasion from time to time, and be by
yourself.**

▶ *Common kitchens* — the next step outside
the intimacy of each others' rooms, and the
chance to broaden your circle during the
spectacularly social events of cooking and
eating. This is not as good for slagging
people off because you are never quite sure
who might feed the information back to the
people concerned.

▶ *Common-room bars in halls* — cosier and
less noisy than union bars. They often have
TV sets and sofas, and are sometimes
equipped with ping-pong tables or bar
billiards, which help the social interaction
along.

A TYPICAL STUDENT KITCHEN:

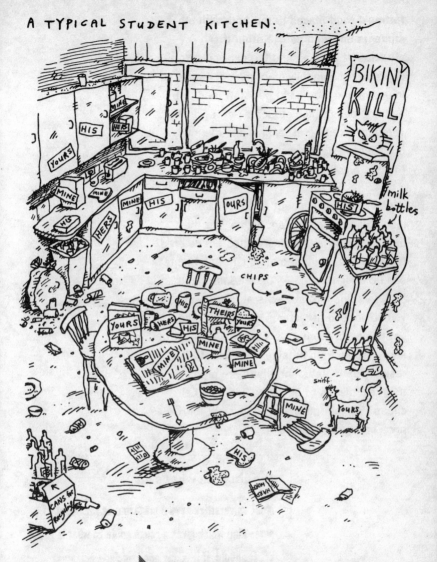

Student Union bars — these tend to be large, noisy, crowded, popular, and very busy. Some have live bands, competing with TV and juke boxes. The drink is usually cheap, the atmosphere smoky and studenty.

Pubs — good places to mix both with other students and with people other than students, if you can find the right pub. You can also occasionally meet members of staff in unguarded moments, but staff tend to try and find pubs which students don't frequent. The drinks can be expensive and the music dull, but the occasional Karaoke or Quiz Night is a good laugh.

Clubs — be picky about where you go. In many places the 'student nights' are the best. Normally all musical tastes are catered for, with DJs taking requests ('Theme Nights' can be a nightmare — 70s or 'Soul'). You tend to bump into students at clubs who you've noticed at lectures or tutorials and get talking to them. It is a great way to get to know people from outside your hall of residence; and student nights are probably the 'key' places to be seen. Beer can be cheap (80p per pint) and an all-night entry price can be around £2–4.

Finding out what's on

Most universities have a magazine or rag sheet of some kind which gives a rough guide to what is going on. It should, if it is any good, include cinemas, theatres, raves, club nights, and discos.

MONEY

The hard graft of it A leap into having to manage your own money is an almost inevitable consequence of college life. Yes, you may have been managing some of it already, but your involvement now is likely to be of a different order:

- even if you get a grant, this will cover only 50% of what the government thinks you need to live on. For the rest, you will have to take out a student loan, earn some money, or rely on your parents

- it is virtually impossible not to end your undergraduate years in debt — to your parents, to your friends, to the bank, or to the student loan fund. The government wants it that way, so don't worry too much

- you need to try and work out some kind of rough budget, if only to give you an idea of priorities and the amount of money you may or may not be able to spend (see below)

- less and less of students' money is coming from grants, and more and more is coming from loans — and most of the money that is available is means tested

Action

➤ by May of the year you are starting college you need to have applied for your grant

➤ in March of that year, find out where your local education authority office is, the one that deals with grants (and the one for where you think you will be living on 30 June of that year). Your local county council (which is in the telephone book) will give you the information

➤ get hold of *Student Grants and Loans: a Brief Guide for Higher Education Students* published by the Department for Education. It's free and should be available at schools, universities, libraries, and local education authorities

➤ ask them to send you the appropriate forms (you can collect them if you want to), fill them in, and return them

➤ if you think you will need a Christmas job, you will have to apply in September/October for places like Sainsbury's, Marks & Spencer, and the Post Office

The experiences of others

❝ **Money, or rather the lack of it, is definitely the most stressful part of university life,** even without the drinking and smoking. Having to decide whether you have enough money to buy a stamp or a pint of milk is a nightmare. On teaching practice, there are lots of materials that you have to have which add up to a substantial amount each week.

A lot depends on the kind of person you are. Sue's parents both work in banks and she says they'd rather she committed murder than went into debt. So far she has managed to keep to her budget, though she had some money saved from her holiday job. The only thing that is getting me through this term is the fact that I have a job to go to at Christmas. Otherwise the prospect would be enough to make the average student commit suicide.

It's unfair that residence fees vary so much from college to college and from university to university. At one university the residence fees are £200 per term, at another they are £700. This puts some students at a disadvantage before they even start. Taking out a student loan is easy, perhaps too easy, as you are not made fully aware of how much the repayments are going to be and what kind of commitment you are actually making. An overdraft from the bank means that unless you can pay it off during the holidays, you have even less to live off during the following term. The banks here are orientated towards getting students' accounts and it's very easy to get an overdraft facility. **9**

❻ There was a group of people who had better financial backing than me and persuaded me to go "clubbing", something I hadn't experienced in my home town. It cost £10–15 a night. Needless to say, at the end of my first term, my first overdraft appeared and by the end of my second term, it had risen to £400 and I couldn't afford to go out at all. This might not seem too great a sum, but I had no means of paying it off.

It was easier to find work near college than at home, but even so it took me two weeks of the summer holidays to find two jobs — one working in a factory from 8.30 a.m. till 5 p.m. and the other in the evening from 6.30 p.m. till 10 working as a barmaid in a pub. I worked every day except weekends, and even then I had to do my evening job on Sundays. I carried on until the beginning of term and then I kept on my evening job so that I could pay off my overdraft — but my work definitely suffered. **❾**

....

How do students cope with money?

Student grants were frozen in 1990. As a result it is now inevitable that almost every student will be in debt at the time of graduation.

From a survey of student debts — in 1993 a student graduating from university owed an average of £1,900. This debt included student loans. The problem that students will have to solve is how to borrow this money at minimum cost. The least expensive way of borrowing money is the bank's free overdraft; after that it is probably best to get the maximum student loan. But watch out for Barclaycard and other bits of plastic for which you pay through the nose.

Students always underestimate the amount of money they will need to borrow during their time at university. They think they will be able to pay off their debts from one year to the next by having holiday jobs. This does not work out in practice and the debt gradually accumulates. Men tend to owe more than women and many have a debt of over £1,000 by the end of their first year.

Some groups of students, such as students with a disability, may be eligible for disabled students' allowances. The National Union of Students is a good source for general information on this as is Skill: The National Bureau for Students with Disabilities (336 Brixton Rd, London, SW9 7AA — tel. 071 274 0565).

Grants and loans At the moment, tuition fees for recognized courses (dance and theatre may be discretionary) tend to be paid — but you need to check with your local authority.

Local authority grants for living expenses are means tested on parental contribution if you are dependent, and on your own earnings

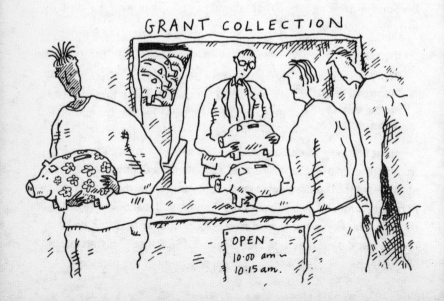

if you are independent (25 or over; married for two years prior to application — but your spouse's income will be means tested; or self-supporting for three years prior to starting the course).

Student loans are available at any time during the academic year. You need proof that you are a student and there are various types of forms to fill in depending on whether this is a first loan or not and which year you are in at university. You can apply only once during an academic year. You will not be asked to begin paying back your loan until the April of the year after you have finished your course, providing that your income is more than 85% of national average earnings. The interest you pay on the loan is linked to inflation. Most borrowers pay it back in sixty instalments over five years.

Money tips for new students

▶ apply for your local authority grant well in advance so that you know it is safe and sound

▶ try and find out any other allowances and benefits that you may be able to claim. Contacting your student union or university business officer may help here

▶ work out a rough budget for yourself (see below). There are some things that you have to have — food, books, and some clothes; but there are other things which, when you begin to feel the pinch, you might be able to do without — ten pints of beer a night, five packets of fags, the odd E tablet. That's not to say that you don't need money for 'play', but just that this is an area that might be easier to ease up on if you're strapped for cash

▶ negotiate with your parents what they are willing to offer you (if anything: many parents may be having a hard financial time themselves, and the occasional parent is simply mean). Money, phonecards, tickets for travelling home, food supplies when they visit, are the sort of things you could discuss

▶ when you arrive at university, collect your grant cheque (different universities arrange this in different ways)

- decide which bank you want to bank with from criteria based on the best deals for interest-free overdrafts and the interest you will have to pay if you go beyond your free overdraft limit

- for most subjects, unless you are rich, don't buy books before you get to university because there is usually a thriving second-hand market. Reading lists given out are not always ideal

- it's best to talk to last year's students (but beware, even second-year students are into the 'market place' mentality, and may try to sell you out-of-date editions at a so-called 'bargain basement' price)

- you do own expensive items, even if you think of yourself as broke — think what it would cost to replace your music centre, tapes, CDs, clothes, books, if they got stolen. It does happen all the time and we often forget to lock our doors. You can see if your parents will insure these items under their household insurance (it needs a special clause to be written in), or you can take out your own insurance. There are special rates for students — but shop around

- banks try and persuade you not to spread your borrowing over different sources — probably sound advice but often impossible. This at least helps you keep track of things (but maybe your reason for spreading the debt is so that you can forget all about it!)

- if you are getting into financial trouble, seek advice and don't just accept sinking under it all. Student unions, the NUS, and/or colleges, usually have someone who will advise you. Being in debt is a fact of life for students nowadays — the government has forced this on to them. It is nothing to be ashamed of, but none of us likes it

- getting a job (either part-time during term, or in the vacation) will help your finances. You will need to balance work, play and study as some students who work for money find that this is achieved at the expense of academic work

- don't buy life insurance unless you have a family — though people will try and flog it to you

▶ if you do have anything to save, or want to make the most of your money, deposit accounts or building societies are best. You'll need to get it out at short notice, unless you're loaded with dosh, in which case you don't even need to read this chapter!

More student experiences

'At the end of the first term I was overdrawn and it seemed a huge amount of money — £600. There was no way of paying this back, so I applied for a student loan which is what I shall live off till my next grant cheque comes through. I'm also looking for a job, though the local Job Centre isn't exactly full of them. I don't mind what I do to keep me out of debt: cleaning toilets out in the local restaurant, waitressing, serving in a shop, cleaning windows — anything. The bank has cancelled my overdraft facility, even though they know I will be getting grant cheques for the next three years. I didn't want a student loan this early, but it's the only way I can survive. A loan is the same as being overdrawn, but you're not pressurized to pay it back until after you leave college. I don't ever want another overdraft.

I have not been able to tell my parents of my predicament. I know they wouldn't approve of my actions and they would want to pay off my debts. But as they can't afford to, I don't see the point in worrying them. At least this way I keep their trust.'

'I've tried to avoid a huge financial burden. I've been living in cheap accommodation, drinking less than the average student, not running a car, or a huge collection of Chris de Burgh CDs, eating casseroles with liver instead of meat, and going to Sainsbury's at 5 p.m. to catch the "reduced for quick sale" bargains. Help also came from my flatmate. He has hefty financial support from his parents, as well as a grant (I don't know how they swung it). So he possesses many unheard of luxuries: a microwave, a serious hi-fi with a CD collection to match, a washer/dryer, a colour telly, a remote control video, even an electric toothbrush. One thing this saved me was hundreds of soul-destroying visits to the local launderette (no, not beautiful and not mine). The only thing that remained constantly hungry was the electricity meter.'

RUNNING OUT OF MONEY!

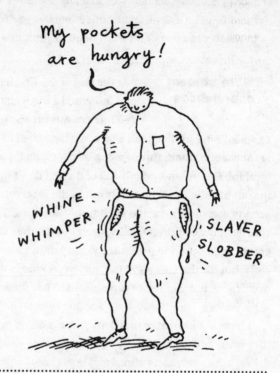

My pockets are hungry!

WHINE WHIMPER

SLAVER SLOBBER

Budgeting

You get your money at the beginning of term — a grant, or what your parents give you, or maybe what you've managed to earn yourself. It will look an enormous sum but it will have to last you until the end of term, and even into the holidays.

How many weeks is that? 8? 10? 12?

Subtract the lump sums you have to pay for the whole term (hall or lodgings, kitchen charges, and so on). Divide what is left over by the number of weeks it has got to last, and that will show you just how little you have to spend each week on everything else.

Don't forget to leave yourself enough to get home again at the end of term!

Essentials for the year

(the costs have to be very rough averages to give
you some idea of budgeting; fill in your costs when
you know them)

	£ p.a.
Accommodation/hall/apartment	1,500
Transport	160
Food	650
Fuel	90
Books and equipment	250
Stationery (pens, paper)	90
Clothes	160
Other (e.g. aspirin, tampons)	80
Contraceptives (get free from your doc!)	
TOTAL	2,980

which represents **£993 per term**
or (with 3 terms of 10 weeks each) **£ 99 per week**

If you are on a full grant, you will get **£2,040** for the
academic year 1994/95 (£2,560 in London).
The year's student loan is £1,150 (£1,375 in London).
This adds up to £3,190 (£3,935 in London) which
doesn't leave much for the so-called 'non-essentials'
over a year.

Note: The Council Tax is a wonderful piece of
government madness.

* you don't have to pay it if you are living in a hall
  of residence

* you don't have to pay it if you are living in a house
  where all the other occupants are students

* you do have to pay it if you are living in a house
  where any other member of that household is not
  a student (though in this case there may be some
  reduction for students)

Suggested non-essentials for the year

	£ p.a.
Telephoning	70
Booze, entertainment, cinema, etc.	680
Insurances	60
TV (must get a licence), CDs, etc.	60
Holiday travel	270
Presents and other incidentals	250
TOTAL	1,390

which represents **£463 per term**
or (with 3 terms of 10 weeks each) **£46 per week**

**To which add fags — if you must, a pack a day
— this will set you back a further £800 a year.**

Jan gets a grant and a loan for living equal to
about **£1,000 per term**:

	£ per term
College accommodation (which includes heating, lighting and one meal)	500
All other food (incl. coffee, milk, etc.) at £3.50 per day	245
Books (expense is mainly early on)	70
Stationery (pens, paper, etc.)	30
Transport to and from home	40
Transport during term	30
TOTAL	£915

**This means Jan has all of £8.50 per week to
spend on non-essentials like clothes, telephone,
cinema, and drinks.**

CHAPTER 5

FRIENDS

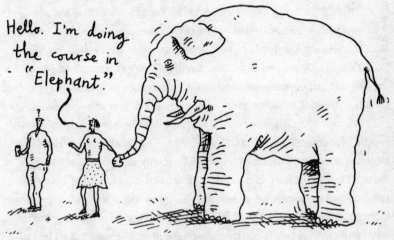

Hello. I'm doing the course in "Elephant."

SOME USEFUL ADVICE FOR MAKING FRIENDS — FIND SOMETHING YOU HAVE IN COMMON.

Susie from Reading University

❝When you first arrive at college you walk around with a permanently cultured, friendly and open smile on your face, hoping that someone will come and talk to you. They don't, so you have to go and talk to them. It's easy to make friends because everyone is as desperate as you are to get to know people. The trouble is, you are usually so desperate at the beginning that you will talk to anyone at all, and after you've got to know a few people, the chances are you will find that the first person you met, you now cannot bear but it's impossible to get rid of them. So it's best to tread carefully before declaring undying friendship to the first person who smiles kindly in your direction. You are meeting so many new people that there is bound to be someone you like, but it does take time.❞

❝ On my very first day at university I felt that I was the most lonely living being. My "contact" didn't show up and it seemed to me that I had made the biggest mistake of my life. After a short period of contemplating suicide, I decided to venture downstairs in the hope of finding someone whom I could befriend. It didn't take long to bump into another bewildered student who appeared to be "contactless" too. We quickly (and eagerly) made friends and decided to have coffee together.

As the weeks grew into months, we became very close friends — probably because we hadn't met many other people we liked. I often wonder what would have happened if we hadn't spoken to one another that day. By the end of the first month of term, everyone had paired off into little twosomes, all of whom were craving new and more exciting friends. The pairs, however, remained in the face of fear of being alone.

Then as the atmosphere relaxed a little, friendships began to drift and people became less tolerant and less polite to one another. New friendships began to form, and I became friends with a girl living opposite me, even though I still spent most of my time with my first friend. A lot of jealousy resulted and the atmosphere became tense, with social activities becoming a nightmare. Both my new friend and I are a few years older than most of the other students, and we found this tiresome and immature. I knew I had to let someone down, but I also felt trapped and in need of broadening my social horizons.

Fortunately, I began working in a pub several times a week. This gave me the opportunity to break out of my social impasse and mix with others. I do think that students should be less insecure and a bit more adventurous when it comes to making friends. ❞

❝ Believe me, by the end of the first week you will be fed up with asking people's names and where they come from (this is where a good knowledge of geography, or a map of the UK comes in handy). But don't be put off so-called "polite conversation" — it has its uses.

It's probably easier making friends in halls or college houses, as you all live close together. On my first night, I had eight people in my room, all chatting and watching me unpack. Most of them were brilliant, but I did seem to spend a good deal of the first term trying to undo false friendships.

Friendships at college change constantly. Sometimes groups emerge, but most people are quite happy to sit and talk with anyone, into the early hours of the morning. A great way to meet people and make loads of friends is to become involved in societies, committees, and unions. You are beginning a fresh period in your life, and trying not to make the same mistakes twice! On the other hand, there are bound to be moments when you feel insecure, because you never really know another person until a few years have passed. People tend to try and hide their bad ways and annoying habits, though these nearly always come out sooner or later. No one is perfect, and it's best not to arrive with the expectation of instantly finding your "bosom buddy". ◗

Ian from Edinburgh University

◖ My perception of university was very romantic, probably from watching too many black and white films set in Oxford or Cambridge — though my university was Edinburgh. I lived in hall, and in the third week of term I formed a very close relationship with a chemistry student. He was my first boyfriend. I felt love for the first time and it really knocked me for six. I couldn't bear being away from him — so much so that I unofficially shared his room. Although he wasn't my usual type, he was very understanding and affectionate and reciprocated my feelings. I would miss lectures and tutorials to be with him, and spend all day in bed, though he wouldn't miss any of his lectures.

Things snowballed quickly out of my control. I developed cystitis (surprise, surprise), and had to take even more time away from work. By the second half of the term, I was getting letters from my tutors and directors of studies, complaining about missed lectures and late coursework. To my chagrin, my boyfriend, instead of supporting me, was furious with me for not having done the work. Like all fairy tales, it didn't last but I suppose it was a character building experience. ◗

*Paul from
Southampton
University*

'Ah, relationships, my life-long obsession, my reason for not getting down to studying — and yet, strangely, the least successful area of my life. I am the kind of person that magazines base their agony columns on. I have had several "affairs" but all without the knowledge of the other person!

Everyone I know has felt deeply involved in my personal traumas over the past year. '

' My problems at university lay mainly in my personal relationships. Leaving home was particularly hard for me, as I left behind some very close friends, including my closest male friend who went off to Cambridge to study English, and my good friend Jane who went to Coventry.

The friends I have here are a mixed bunch of individuals who aren't necessarily the ones I would have picked if I had had more choice. '

*Deborah from
Oxford University*

*Bridget from
Swansea University*

'There's such a build-up before you go to university: about these being the best years of your life, the golden years, when you will make your best friends. After a few weeks, I thought, "Ummh, I've had better times, and my friends at home are just as good as the ones I'm making here." '

**The different types which exist in universities are amazing. Students should be students, with no distinctions between creed, class, or colour — an amorphous mass recognizable by their radical ideas about everything, their poverty, their politics, and their love of cheap ale. But in fact, there are as many different types as there are colours of Smarties in a packet.

Coming from a private school and a middle-class background, I imagined people like me would be in the majority, but I did not expect to come up against the blatant élitism that is predominant in some universities. Having said that, I'll get off my soap box.**

Lizzy from Durham University

John from Liverpool University

I didn't really settle down at university until the summer term of my first year. It was probably something to do with my male reserve. The first few weeks were definitely the worst. Week zero, as it was ominously called at some universities, was one long panic attack. Nobody wants to spend their first week alone, and everybody follows the advice given in authoritative books about making friends, which is usually pretty standard and predictable. Apparently, one is meant to run beaming through any open door, clutching a coffee mug. Quite how those on the receiving end are meant to unpack their luggage while letting in a queue of strangers wanting to borrow some Gold Blend is never made clear. I had barely got over the shock of having only one electrical socket outlet when my room was invaded by people I didn't know. My preconceived, melodramatic farewell to my parents was reduced to a flippant, "Oh well, see you around sometime," under the gaze of my new-found "friends".

❝ I had to leave my boyfriend, who had just become my fiancé, two days earlier on his 18th birthday. I still see him regularly, we've only been apart for one weekend, so nothing has really changed in my relationship with him. It's just been altered to accommodate the different circumstances. Now it's hours of phoning, writing, and travelling, instead of just walking into a room to be with one another. OK, so it's tough, but I think we'll survive. ❞

Let's be enemies.

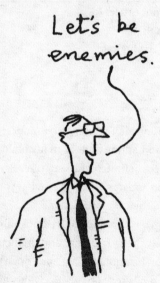
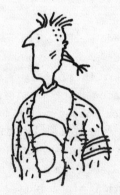

CHAPTER SIX

SEX&RELATIONSHIPS

Being at college doesn't mean that you
automatically have to take out membership of the
sex subculture, but if you do join — either
wholeheartedly or occasionally — **be prepared!**

A lecture note for students on sex

▶ on any one night in the world, with 2.5 billion
sexually active people, there are at least
200,000,000 doing it (to say nothing of those
who are doing it during the day!)

▶ this activity will result (every night, mind you)
in 900,000 conceptions, at least half of them
unplanned, 350,000 sexual infections, and will
lead to 100,000 abortions

Some People

Some people like sex more than others —
You seem to like it a lot.
There's nothing wrong with being innocent
  or high-minded
But I'm glad that you're not.

Wendy Cope

❛Most people I slept with were friends, so seduction was more a question of circumstance than of verbal dexterity. After drinking far too much, you'd find yourself in a semi-coma on the sofa with one of your numerous acquaintances. If it was five in the morning and you lived across town, rather than trek home, you would slope off with them. A lot of sex at university is to do with laziness, vanity, and the inability to say no owing to the fact that you have drunk too much.❜

❛Us students are pretty shy about making sexual advances. People move in tight social circles and any romantic developments are prime gossip fodder. Since sex with a stranger requires even more confidence and bravery than sex among one's own, most people eventually choose bed partners within their own clique. Me and my male friends were far more sexually timid and frustrated than our female counterparts.❜

❛Male students tend to be amazingly filthy in their personal habits, and after spending the night with one boy who hadn't changed his sheets in three years, I developed an aversion for sex with scholars. Our relationship was short-lived and had been the product of "fuck a fresher" week. Freshers are easy prey, feeling (as I did) lost, lonely and socially leprous — a powerful incentive to jump straight into the arms of the nearest lecher. I can't remember when we first snogged, but we split up when he projectile vomited a nasty mixture of beer, chips and gravy all over the corridor of my hall.❜

❛I had this boyfriend and we were sleeping together, so I applied for a place in the same city as him. Even though I didn't get the grades, I did get in where I wanted. At the beginning of the first term, we travelled up together and arrived together at my hall of residence. I didn't notice at the time, but it must have looked a bit strange — every one else being with their parents.

We had been going out since we were 15, and before he went on to his own college he asked if we could get engaged. We had talked about it and agreed it would happen at some point. Now we talked in a light-hearted way about getting married as well.

After Easter, for some reason I came back to college on my own. Towards the end of the journey, the man sitting next to me started a conversation. He seemed nice, carried my cases, and invited me to see a play he was in. I didn't think much of it at the time, and although I quite liked him, it was all a bit tenuous. But it did start me thinking about John.

I began to see what my life would be like if I stayed with him. John was in his third and final year, and after college he would probably return home and do accountancy. I could visualize the sort of house we would live in — even the fireplace, and it wasn't what I wanted. When John got back to college, I ended the relationship. I hadn't wanted to do it then. He was just about to take his finals. But I couldn't see him and not say anything. It was awful.⁹

⁶**I'm lucky, in my group there is no pressure at all to have sex.** There are fifteen of us altogether who are friends. Everyone is someone I could spend time with, and when I go to a party I make a bee line for one of them. There are four or five among them whom I do feel closer to, but we seem to manage to give each other space, to do our own thing and have a good laugh, without any pressure to have sex. It's not that I'm against sex in any moral way; I've just not felt the urge yet with anyone I've met.⁹

⁶**I remember when one of my friends said that she was having a lesbian affair.** We were on a train together, which had given her the chance to let out all sorts of secrets that I wasn't sure I actually wanted to know. My reaction to the last confession was, I suppose, initially tainted with a little shock, even disgust. Not that I haven't at times felt strongly attracted to my girlfriends, but this friend had so many emotional problems and confusions that this did not seem like a strong decision which made her happier about herself as a result. It seemed instead like another desperate attempt to find herself, and I really didn't want to have to deal with this side of her character. After all, I had never encouraged her to confide in me in this way.

I suppose I was fearful that having involved me in her worries, she'd then expect me to take it one step further and become her lover. At that moment, sitting in a grotty railway carriage, I found the whole idea a bit sordid. I hope I said the right things and didn't make her feel awful, as it was a big thing to confide in someone. But I didn't want to reciprocate and tell her personal things about myself. I was aware, however, that my immediate reaction hadn't been exactly politically correct. She rather froze up after that, and I decided that if it happened to me again I would try harder to understand — and not just have a hysterical reaction to the word "lesbian".**9**

6 What is wrong about a sexual and emotional relationship between two people who are committed to an equal partnership, with love and respect at its core — just because they happen to be both men or both women? At school I learnt that sex should only take place between a man and a woman within marriage, that masturbation is wrong, and that homosexuality is unnatural. I was aware that most young people go through a phase of being attracted to members of the same sex, but I knew I was different and that this attraction for me was far too strong and too keenly felt to be dismissed as a teenage "phase".

As an undergraduate, I realized that I couldn't go on deceiving myself. The most difficult part was hearing myself say "I'm gay" to another person (in my case, my doctor). I had never discussed an emotional problem with a doctor before; I thought it might be regarded as a trivial matter compared with the problems of other patients. I can't put into words how relieved I was to talk to someone about it. I'd kept so much fear, so much confusion and worry inside me for so long. I also read some books about homosexuality and I found them comforting and reassuring.

I don't see my sexuality as a "choice" or a "preference": it is simply what I am. The only choice I have is to accept my homosexuality, and therefore myself, or to deceive myself and those around me by pretending to be heterosexual. I have told two close friends (both heterosexual) that I'm gay. One of them said that it wouldn't make any difference to our friendship and he still cares about me — in fact I think this has brought us closer together. My other friend was shocked, though he said this wouldn't change our relationship. But as he appears to think that we don't need to talk about it ever again, this has created a distance between us.

I can't change what I am, for anyone. Coming to terms with my sexuality is a painful, difficult and lonely process, but I like to think that I am moving towards a much greater acceptance of myself.⁹

⁶**University was a period of more or less uninterrupted and much wanted celibacy for me.** The sexual scene there was very black and white. People were either knee deep in long-term relationships, or they never seemed to have sex at all. There was no lighthearted snogging because people were too preoccupied with appearing cool, or too good a friend to be an option. Anyhow, most of the decent girls seemed to have been snapped up within a week of arrival.⁹

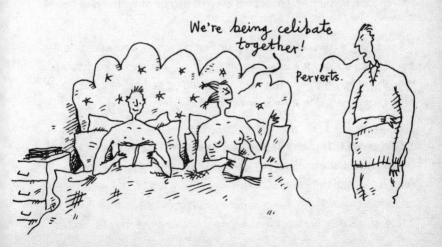

❝A friend of mine, someone I would bump into from time to time, came up to me in the street and told me he was gay. To start with I thought he was joking. Then I thought, "What does he want from me?" But he said he'd already told all his close friends, and his brother, and now he was starting to tell people he saw now and then. Interestingly, he hadn't told his parents. It was quite out of the blue, because he was now in the third year and I knew he'd been out with a couple of girls. He seemed really relieved and happy to be telling me; and was into discussing who he fancied (not me!), and how his love life was going.❞

❝Many of the boys I know are really homophobic and make cutting remarks about gays. They really seem to be uncomfortable with the idea of homosexuality. I'm in a drama group and several of the guys are gay. I was walking with a gay guy and a straight guy to lectures one day, and we were talking about the play we were doing and about one of the characters in the play who is gay. It was awful, because my straight friend started saying, "Oh my God, how can anyone be gay?" The girls seem much more accepting. The men all seem threatened by it, which surprises me.

The campus has a gay and lesbian "rights" officer who has been getting a lot of hassle from some of the students in the student newspaper. Somehow, I expected everyone to be more tolerant here.❞

❝Snogging with a student at your own university never seemed like much of an option. It's a bit like snogging on your own front doorstep, though I did try my hand (and mouth, including half an hour munching on a flaccid penis) at it once or twice.❞

❝The great thing about coming to university was being able to be myself. I'd always been attracted to other women — but could only feel comfortable showing it here.❞

What degree would you get in contraception?

Please answer the following questions:

1 *How many hours after having unprotected intercourse can you still use 'emergency' contraception?*

— 2 hours   — 48 hours

— 12 hours   — 72 hours

— 24 hours   — 5 days

2 *From which of the following can you get emergency contraception?*

— students' union

— local chemist

— your own GP

— any GP

— family planning clinic

— local hospital accident and emergency department

3 *Under which of the following circumstances should you consider using emergency contraception?*

— you (she) are (is) on the pill, and you (she) take(s) it four hours late
— you are using the withdrawal method but you (he) fail(s) to come out (stuck, forgets, gets carried away!)
— the condom splits, drops off (just isn't there when you think it should be!)
— you (he) ejaculate(s) somewhere near, but not in, her (your) vagina
— you are having unprotected sex in what you think is the safe period
— you had unprotected sex a week ago

4 *At what speed does sperm leave the end of the penis during ejaculation?*

— 5 miles an hour
— 13 miles an hour
— 28 miles an hour
— 39 miles an hour
— 56 miles an hour

5 *How long does the average sperm hang out in the average vagina (and/or environs)?*

— 4 hours   — 4 days
— 12 hours   — a week
— 36 hours

6 *Which of the following are reliable methods of contraception?*

— the contraceptive sponge
— the Femidom (the female condom)
— withdrawal
— the 'safe' period
— condoms
— the cap
— spermicidal jelly
— the pill

7 *Which is the best method of contraception for students to use?*

— non-penetrative sex
— condoms
— the cap
— the pill
— 'NO'
— an IUD
— withdrawal
— the 'safe' period
— the Femidom
— the contraceptive sponge

8 *You are a male and a female student together for one night and you have unprotected sex. What are the chances of her getting pregnant?*

— 10%
— 20%
— 30%
— 40%
— 80%
— 100%

On Planet Percy males ejaculate one large sperm which strolls across to the female, knocks politely and asks if he may come in.

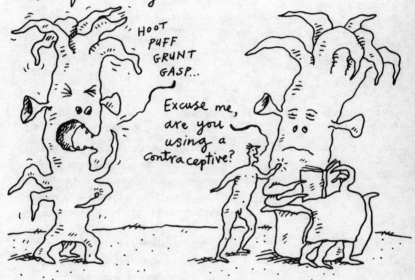

HOOT
PUFF
GRUNT
GASP...

Excuse me, are you using a contraceptive?

9 *Which of the following are true about the pill?*

— it makes you fat
— it's 100% safe
— it helps protect you against sexually transmitted diseases (STDs)
— it causes cancer
— it makes you infertile if you take it for a long time
— you shouldn't smoke and be on the pill
— it makes you depressed
— it makes it more likely that you will have sex

10 *A man who is HIV negative has vaginal intercourse once with a woman who is HIV positive. What are the chances of his catching the AIDS virus?*

— 1 in 5
— 1 in 20
— 1 in 50
— 1 in 100
— 1 in 1000

Answers

1 *72 hours* — so don't wake your doctor at 2 a.m. — she or he may not thank you for it, particularly as she or he may have been making love. If it happens on Saturday night, Monday morning is early enough. However, if the receptionist won't give you an emergency appointment, don't take 'no' for an answer. It may help to explain what it's about (so don't be embarrassed) — but you shouldn't have to.

2 *You can get it from:*
▸ your own GP
▸ any GP
▸ family planning clinic
▸ local hospital accident and emergency department

Sometime in the future, perhaps, you will be able to get it from the local chemist, but not yet alas.

3a *You should get emergency contraception if:*

▪ you are using the withdrawal method but you (he) fail(s) to come out. **It takes only a minute amount of sperm to get pregnant — each 2ml of the stuff contains 20,000,000 or so sperm — enough to populate the whole of Australia at one go.**

▪ the condom splits or drops off — the same applies, a little sperm goes a long way.

▪ you are having unprotected sex in what you think is the safe period. Unless you are willing to monitor your periods, temperature, and vaginal mucus changes, throughout each month, there is no such thing as an absolutely 'safe' period — it's just a less 'unsafe' period.

3b *You don't have to rush off for emergency contraception if:*

▪ you (she) are (is) on the pill, but take(s) it 4 hours late — the pill still works perfectly well under these circumstances. If you are less than 12 hours late in taking the pill, there is nothing to worry about. Later than that, you need to start taking the pill again and use some other forms of contraception for 7 days. (This applies only to the combined pill: see Chapter 8.)

▪ you (he) ejaculate(s) somewhere near, but not in, her (your) vagina. Men should not squirt too much semen around, but, on the other hand, it doesn't survive very well outside the vagina. 'Virgin' births are very rare — with only one confirmed case that we know of!

▪ you had unprotected sex a week ago. If you got the answer to Question 1 right, you should know about this one (it's too late; if your period doesn't come on time, it's off to the chemist, or your doctor, for a pregnancy test kit).

4 **28 miles an hour is the average, and don't ask how it was measured (trapped by a speed camera?). No fines for over 30 m.p.h. though**.

5 Most sperm are fragile little things and die off quickly. However, they can last for up to 4 days — and watch out for the 7-day lunatic fringe.

6 Depends on what you mean by 'reliable'. There is 'reliable' for not getting pregnant, and 'reliable' for not getting a sexually transmitted disease (STD).

Condoms

- good for not getting pregnant. 98 women out of 100, using condoms for a year every night, will not get pregnant.
- also the best protection against STDs.

The Femidom (the female condom)

- Like the male equivalent, it is good for not getting pregnant, and protects against STDs — but oh dear, it can be a bit noisy!

The Pill

- 'the best' for not getting pregnant. If used carefully, the combined pill is virtually 100% safe. It offers no protection against STDs though.

Spermicidal Jelly, the Contraceptive Sponge, Withdrawal and the Safe Period

- None of these are very reliable methods if you don't want to get pregnant, and they don't protect you from catching STDs either. But they are all better than nothing. How often you get pregnant using one of these methods very much depends on how careful you are, as well as the method itself.

The Cap (or diaphragm)

- fairly good protection against pregnancy. 96 women out of 100, using the cap every night for a year, will not get pregnant.
- some protection against STDs.

An IUD

- not recommended (see Chapter 8)

7   There is no best overall method — only a best individual method for you and your partner. As you may not want to go on saying 'no' indefinitely, you had better sort something out in advance for when you want to say 'yes'. If you're an optimist, you'll be pleased at all the different choices; if you're a pessimist, you'll feel that all of them have their drawbacks. You have to end up being a pragmatist and choose one of the methods. The best method for you will depend on the type of relationship you are involved in, your previous experience, and your anxieties. What is best in one relationship, may not be best in another.

8   It depends on where you (she) are (is) in your (her) menstrual cycle. The egg is normally released about 14 days before the next period is due and the chances of getting pregnant at this time are 30%. For about 5 to 10 days either side of this time, the chances are 20%; and for the rest of the cycle (what little there is of it left) the chances are 0 to 10% — but don't rely on that '0'.

9   *The truth about the pill:*

▶   *it makes you fat:* **NOT TRUE.** A small percentage of women put on a few pounds, but you can nearly always find a pill that doesn't cause this problem.

▶   *it's 100% safe:* **TRUE.** If it is taken properly, it is almost 100% effective in stopping you getting pregnant.

▶   *it helps protect you against* **STDs: NOT TRUE.** It does not protect you against STDs so it might be a good idea to use the pill and condoms.

▶   *it causes cancer:* **NOT TRUE AND TRUE.** The pill reduces the risk of ovarian and uterine (womb) cancer, but if you take it for 5 years or more there is probably a small increased risk of cervical cancer (which is very rare anyhow). It's therefore a good idea to have regular cervical smears. The other cancer that may be affected by taking the pill is breast cancer. We still don't know exactly how breast cancer risk is affected if you take the pill when you are young — some of the evidence is conflicting; but there is some to suggest that if you take the pill for 5 years or more, there may be a small increased risk.

- *it makes you infertile if you take it for a long time:* **NOT REALLY TRUE.** The pill does not make you infertile. However, if you have taken it for many years and you stop it to try and get pregnant, it might take a bit longer than usual (up to 2 years).

- *you shouldn't smoke and be on the pill:* **TRUE.** It's best not to smoke anyway (OK, we know you won't listen to preaching about this), but apart from all the other nasty things fags do, if you smoke and take the pill you have a slightly increased chance of getting a heart attack or a blood clot. (Admittedly, it's a very small risk as risks go.)

- *it makes you depressed:* **TRUE AND NOT TRUE.** Most people do not get depressed on the pill, but a small percentage do and if it happens to you, the best thing is to change pills and see if you can find one that suits you. There are over 10 different combinations.

- *it makes it more likely that you will have sex:* **NOT TRUE.** Whether people have sex or not doesn't seem to depend on whether they are on the pill or not. Most studies indicate that it depends on immediate circumstances: the attraction of the partner, the time of night, alcohol, privacy, bed available, and so on.

10 **The answer is between 1 in 100 and 1 in 1000 — and it is probably towards the 1 in 1000 end.** The chances are better than in Russian roulette — but why take the risk when you can (a) do lots of sexy things without having intercourse and (b) use a condom. When an HIV negative woman has sex with an HIV positive man, the risk swings to the 1 in 100 end. Therefore women have a higher risk of catching the AIDS virus from men than men have from women.

Your degree:

If you scored 80% to 100% you get a first

If you scored 70% to 80% you get a 2.1

If you scored 60% to 70% you get a 2.2

If you scored 50% to 60% you get a third

Below 50% is a failure and you'll have to retake —
and no sex with anyone till you pass

CHAPTER 8

'I promise I won't come...

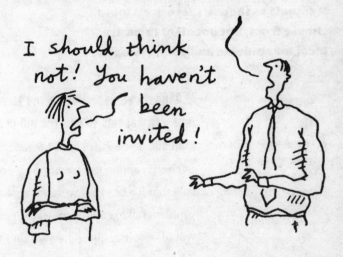

I should think not! You haven't been invited!

...must be the most unreliable method around.'

Most students will want to have sex during their time at university, and certainly most will not want to get pregnant, so you will have to suss out the contraceptive scene and use something, or get your partner to. The two most commonly used methods of contraception among students are the condom and/or the pill. But a survey showed that 30 to 50 per cent of students having sex for the first time didn't take any precautions.

The methods of contraception available are condoms, the combined pill, the progesterone-only pill, the diaphragm or cap, spermicides, the female condom (the Femidom), the 'safe' period with fertility awareness, withdrawal, progesterone injections, and the IUD. One or two other methods are being developed, but at the moment these are all variations on a theme rather than anything truly revolutionary. **It sounds as though there are a lot to choose from, but not all of them are ideal for students and young people.**

❝ Almost everyone I've talked to at my university seems to use the pill or a condom. Some girls I spoke to saw the subject of contraception as an emotional one; others said that if a boy they were seeing had a problem talking about contraception, they would seriously question what they were doing with him.

There was also the feeling that if you discuss it too much, it reduces sex to a purely biological level. ❞

A 'Quickie's Guide' To Contraception

	Condoms	Pill	Cap	Sponge/ Withdrawal	Non—Penetrative sex
For one night stands	Excellent	OK	OK	Better than nothing!	Excellent
To avoid STDs	Excellent	No good	OKish	Useless	OK
For long term relationships	Excellent	Excellent	Good	Not reliable	OK (as long as non-penetration lasts!)
If you must smoke	Excellent	Some risks	Good	Not reliable	Excellent
Just in case you get the urge	Excellent	OK	OK	Not reliable	Excellent
Neither has had sex before	Excellent	Excellent	Not so easy	Not reliable	Excellent
He's had sex before	Excellent	OK	Not so easy	Not reliable	Excellent
She's had sex before	Excellent if she can get it on	OK	OK	Not reliable	Excellent
You want to end the relationship	JUST DON'T DO IT — THERE ARE MORE UNWANTED PREGNANCIES AT THE BEGINNING AND END OF RELATIONSHIPS				

Emergency contraception from the user's view

'Absence, if it means abstinence, has its problems. We were so frustrated by weekends that when we did see one another, things tended to get out of hand. The first weekend ended in an unfortunate and all-too-avoidable accident in contraception. We got carried away and used nothing — fun at the time but a disaster. I had to take the "morning after" pill, and had to get it from a somewhat moralistic GP who didn't show a glimmer of humour or sympathy. To my surprise, I was fine. No sickness, no nausea, no nothing.'

'I was lucky to discover the "morning after" pill wasn't literally that! It was forty-eight hours before I managed to get it. I thought you could only get that pill from a family planning clinic. I tried two, and they were both crap because there was no one there at the time who could prescribe it. Finally, in desperation, I went to my own GP, and it turned out not only that he could give it to me, but that any GP could have done. If only I had known.

My GP is a really nice guy — oldish, but he didn't turn on the moralistic bit at all. He was incredibly reassuring after all my haring around, and informed me that the emergency pill works up to seventy-two hours after the "accident". I had to take two pills immediately, and then two more twelve hours later. They made me feel as sick as anything, but I managed not to vomit. He said to come back if I did throw up, as the pills might not get absorbed and I'd need to take some more. When my friend took them, she had a really bad time. She couldn't stop vomiting and had to take something else to stop throwing up.'

- it is estimated that 100,000 abortions in the UK could be avoided each year if everyone at risk (because of split condoms and getting carried away) used emergency contraception

Emergency contraception: The facts

- it works for up to 72 hours after the unprotected intercourse occurs

- it is available free from any GP, family planning clinic, or accident and emergency department in a hospital

- it should only be used in emergencies, not as a regular method of birth control

- if you are using it once a month, get yourself to your family doctor or family planning clinic — or one of you should buy some condoms

- the pills contain oestrogen and progesterone at higher doses than the ordinary contraceptive pill

- they work by stopping implantation of a fertilized ovum (egg)

- you take two pills and then two more 12 hours later

- sometimes they make you sick; if you vomit you should take a couple more pills to replace the two you have thrown up

- emergency contraception is 96% effective

- the only other emergency method is to have an intra-uterine device put in, which works for up to 5 days after unprotected intercourse

- emergency contraceptive pills are likely to be available over the counter at the chemist in the future

---

The 'ons' and 'ons' of condoms

A consultant in genito-urinary medicine

❛ Our results suggest a proportion of men have penises sufficiently large to cause difficulties in putting on condoms. For some men, 70mm (a flat width of 2.76 inches) would not be too large. One patient made a video for us to look at. There is no way that that man could have used a standard British condom. ❜

John from Leeds University

'. . . **slippery little beasts. I used to try and put them on myself, but they kept falling off, and we would start laughing and I would lose my erection.** Then I started to worry that I wouldn't get it up again — but she always managed it. She's much better than me at putting them on so I don't lose it and it's great.'

Jane from Edinburgh University

'**I used to worry that they would slip off and get lost inside me,** but it's never actually happened. They're better now that they come in different sizes and shapes. Men's knobs are not all the same by any means.'

Steven from Oxford Brookes University

'I can't use them. I'm sorry, I know I should, but they are the ultimate turn-off. I just can't manage with them on, and it's not for want of trying. So I go in for all the other sexy things that you can do together without running risks. Oral sex, mutual masturbation, touching one another in strange places — all that kind of thing.'

Edward from Leicester University

'**Condoms are a pain in the arse. Fumbling around in the dark can be embarrassing.** I don't carry them regularly, only when I think I'm in with a chance of scoring. I'm happy when a girl gets them out, and I'm interested in trying the female condom. In the past, women have refused to sleep with me because I didn't have any contraception. Maybe it was just because they thought I was ugly.'

Jenny from Plymouth University

'**Condoms are grim but they're good for one-night stands.** Once I'd had sex without a condom, I didn't want to go back to using one. I always carried condoms before I went on the pill. I never found it embarrassing. I'd make a joke about having condoms early in the evening so when it came to having sex it was OK.'

Condoms: The facts

♦ they protect you against pregnancy and STDs and AIDS

♦ they come in different sizes — from minimum British Standard: width 48mm (1.89 inches) and length 160mm (6.2 inches) to a US brand: width 65mm (2.2 inches) and length 220mm (8.66 inches) — so take your pick

♦ they come in different colours

♦ they come in different shapes (flared, contoured, ribbed)

♦ they come in different flavours

♦ they can be bought everywhere

♦ they can be obtained free from any family planning clinic and some family doctors

♦ they can expand 600% — but can get split by a finger nail when putting them on, especially if the penis is too big or the condom too small when rolled up

♦ 2 women in every 100 using condoms every night for a year will get pregnant

♦ they protect women against cancer of the cervix

♦ always use a new one — they don't cost much and second-hand ones don't have quite the same appeal!

How to use condoms

♦ check the 'use by' date — but any old condom is better than none

♦ unwrap carefully — if you have any nails left, make sure you keep them to yourself

♦ put it on your (his) penis once it's up. If it's not erect, wait — but don't comment (it might droop further). You can't get it on to a flaccid, useless bit of flopsy

♦ make sure it gets on before any come comes, as even a drop of semen will contain the odd 100,000 sperm

- put it on the right penis, the right way round, and with the 'roll' bit outwards — this is more difficult than you think

- squeeze the baggy bit at the end as you roll it on (this reduces the bursting rate, though as the average condom is tested to expand 600% you shouldn't have any trouble)

- keep holding the top end on the penis and roll the rest all the way down

- ***HAVE SEX NOW NOW NOW***

- afterwards (even if you haven't had an orgasm) take the condom off carefully while the penis is still semi-erect, making sure you don't spill anything

- tie a knot in the end and discard — but not down the loo. They float and there are already enough of them in the North Sea. The fish are choking on them — an unpleasant way to go

Supercharging your sex life

An enterprising condom salesman did some market research among the oldest profession to see what kind of advice these experts could give on increasing the appeal of condom use. They suggested the following:

1 *Use a contoured or flared condom which has a space at the end of it.*

2 *Put a dollop of lubricating jelly inside the end of the flared or contoured condom (about a quarter filling it).*

3 *Put the condom on your (his) penis and take whatever action you like (masturbation, oral sex, vaginal intercourse). The lubricating jelly spreads the sensations all around the end of your (his) penis, exciting many more nerve ends than usual.*

People on the pill

Sammy at Brunel University

'I'd always joked about being flat-chested and how the pill would give me a cleavage. It certainly did — but it's a bit of a shock to suddenly have bosoms.

I like the freedom the pill gives you, which is hard to give up once you're used to it. It makes sex more natural with more extension of foreplay than if we had to faff around getting the necessary bits of rubber in place before penetration.

The control over my periods is great too. It is nice, after years of being pretty irregular, to know to the day when my period is going to start; and it is light and only lasts a few days.

I started taking the pill when I became involved in a special relationship. Going to the doctor together and remembering to take it every day seemed to bring us closer. It made me feel I was doing it not just for myself, but for both of us.'

Mike at Newcastle University

'The decision to go on the pill is part of the commitment of going out with someone. It means you can have sex whenever you want. And it means never offending your mother with floating condoms in the toilet.

I sometimes worry about what the pill is doing to my girlfriend, and it seems unfair that all the responsibility rests on her. Arranging for her to go on the pill was a bit stressful for us both. Some girls on the pill feel like a slag because having sex becomes easier when the issue of contraception has been dealt with. Another negative point is that if I have a lot of sex and I'm not wearing a condom, it makes my willy sore.'

'I prefer the responsibility of contraception being with the girl. Boys can't remember to do anything, let alone take a pill. It makes my *Jenny at Bangor University* periods less trouble, unless I forget to take it and then it messes them up. When I do forget a pill, I'm rather lazy about using condoms, and then I get anxious about getting pregnant. When I was on one type of pill, it made me really nauseous and gave me premenstrual tension, so I had to change to another one.'

Tammy at Keele University

'I've been on the pill for several years now and have had no real problems with it till recently, when I think it increased my weight problem leaving me feeling bloated, overweight and depressed. However, I still maintain that at my age and in my circumstances, the pill with a condom is the most sensible option. I have never experienced any difficulties with condoms, and the men I have been with seem to find them OK too.'

The 'pros' and 'cons' of the combined pill

*What's **good** about the combined pill:*

- it's the most reliable form of contraception for not getting pregnant

- while on it women have regular periods each month (so there are no anxieties about being late) and the periods tend to be lighter than usual

- it doesn't interfere with making love

- it's not messy

- men like it because they don't have to take any responsibility

*What's **bad** about the combined pill:*

- it doesn't protect you against STDs or AIDS

- you have to remember to take it every day

- some people don't like taking hormones

- there are some minor side-effects

- a very few people get serious problems

- you have to get it from the doctor

The combined pill: The facts

- it is taken 21 out of 28 days

- the two main ingredients are progesterone and oestrogen in different proportions in different makes of pill

- you start it on the first day of a period and you are 'safe' to have sex immediately

- if you miss a pill for less than 12 hours — take it and don't worry

- if you miss a pill for more than 12 hours — take it and use other precautions for 7 days

- minor side-effects include: weight gain, depression, headaches, going off sex, feeling sick, tender breasts, moodiness; most of these disappear after a couple months, but you can always try another make

- taking the pill doesn't mix well with smoking — you can get blood clots (rarely)

- cancer of the ovary and cancer of the uterus (womb) are reduced if you have taken the pill

- long-term use of the pill (more than 5 years) when you are young may result in a slightly increased risk of getting cancer of the breast

- it is taken by about 50% of women students using contraception

People using the cap

Sue at Sheffield University

❝ It's OK, you're in charge, and you're not filling yourself up with hormones; but it does make sex less spontaneous and pinging it in was a bit of a bother — it kept slipping out of my fingers and shooting across the room. ❞

Jo at Hull University

❝ . . . never even considered using it. I thought it was the kind of thing my mother would have got up to. But now I've tried it and found out how easy it is, I can't imagine why everyone doesn't use one. After all, it's just like shoving in a tampon. Sometimes, though, you do need a sense of humour to cope with it.❞

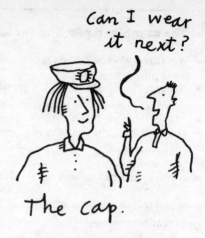

Can I wear it next?

the cap.

Susan from University College, Oxford

❝No thanks. I got pregnant using a cap, though I thought I'd put it in right. It was a nightmare — especially as it was just before my exams.❞

The 'pros' and 'cons' of the cap (diaphragm)

What's good about the cap:

- it is relatively easy to put in

- the woman is in control

- there's no stopping and fiddling in the middle of love-making as there is with a condom

- it is a safe method

- it gives some protection against STDs

What's bad about the cap:

- it has to be fitted

- it has to be checked for correctness of fit every 6 months

- it is a bit messy

- you need to think ahead of time and have it with you

- it is not 100% safe

- it takes a bit of practice to get used to it

- you need access to running water to wash it afterwards

The cap: The facts

- there are several different types (there is also the cervical cap, which some people prefer as it is smaller and can be left in for more than 24 hours)

- the main type comes in eight different sizes

- you need to use a spermicide with it

- you can put it in up to 3 hours before having sex

- it must stay in at least 6 hours after having sex

- it is best stored in a plastic box, not in tissue paper which will become attached

- it can perish and leak in some conditions (hot, humid)

- it is used by about 4–10% of students

Other methods

The Femidom (female condom)

- very effective for prevention of pregnancy and STDs

- a bit like having sex with a plastic bag — and some users say it's noisy

- it fits all sizes of erect penises

- you can buy it over the counter and it doesn't need fitting, but it's expensive for sex every night

Peter from the University of Buckingham

'It was much better than a normal condom, it gave me much more room to move around in, but I found the ring at the bottom a bit annoying.'

Samantha from Liverpool John Moores University

'It was too crinkly, it crackled a lot and made a very off-putting noise.'

The mini-pill/progesterone-only pill (POP)

♦ if you can't take the combined pill, this is an alternative and certainly worth consideration

♦ it consists of progesterone only

♦ it is not as effective at stopping pregnancy as 'the' pill

♦ it is no good if you are scatty about time-keeping, as you have to take it at about the same time every day

♦ other progesterone contraception includes the 'Depo' injection which needs repeating every 3 months, and Norplant (a small device inserted under the skin) which lasts 5 years — but you can get unwanted bleeding between periods

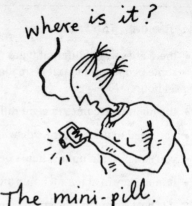

where is it?

The mini-pill.

Intra-uterine device (IUD) or coil

♦ a bit of plastic covered in copper and/or a hormone

♦ it is inserted through the cervix into the uterus

♦ it is not recommended for young women who haven't had children as it increases the risk of getting infected Fallopian tubes, which might affect future chances of getting pregnant

♦ it is a last-resort method for most students

Spermicides

♦ these can be bought over the counter

♦ they are not good used alone but are better than nothing

♦ they help kill the AIDS virus as well as sperm

♦ they are useful as a lubricant

The sponge

♦ a soft, round, plastic sponge impregnated with spermicide that a woman puts into her vagina before sex

♦ it is not as safe as condoms, caps, or the pill (up to 25 out of every 100 women using this method every night will get pregnant in a year)

Natural methods: rhythm and safe period

♦ women ovulate 14 to 16 days before the first day of their next period

♦ this is the time when they are most likely to get pregnant

♦ their temperature goes up slightly and their vaginal mucus changes in character at ovulation

♦ taking your temperature and testing your vaginal mucus, as well as charting the timing of your periods over several months, can tell you which are the more risky times to have intercourse

♦ this can be a reliable method if you have absolutely regular periods, are willing to be obsessional, and have been well taught

Withdrawal

♦ this is not safe, but is better than nothing

♦ it is widely used by everyone

♦ it depends too much on men's self-control — which is not reliable at the best of times!

Just because you're late it doesn't mean you're pregnant, but if you think you could be pregnant because you've taken a risk, then pregnancy is the likely answer and ostrich-like behaviour will not help!

' I'm late . . . '

This old wives method of contraception works by luring the stork into a box with some fish, then putting a sock over its head.

Ah ha...

A 'do it yourself' pregnancy test is what you need first:

- you can buy them from any chemist
- you can use them within 2 days of the 'expected' start of a missed period
- they cost about £5 for two (they usually come in a pack of two)
- they are reliable, and normally if they are positive, you're pregnant
- occasionally they fail to tell you that you're pregnant when you are. If you're still worried, or miss another period, you need to do a second test
- if you're penniless or would prefer someone else to do the test, see a GP or go to a family planning clinic
- some anti-abortion organizations offer free pregnancy testing and 'so-called' non-judgemental counselling, but they are obviously going to have some bias

---

When all else has failed

There is a choice, but for some students it will be a difficult one to make:

- most students who get pregnant by mistake will decide to have an abortion

▶ if you decide to have the baby, and some students do, there will be help at hand. Talk to your parents, your tutor, your GP, or your counsellor. If that is what you want to do, you should go for it, and be supported. You will then have to decide whether to continue with your studies, take time out, or have the baby adopted

The things you need to think about are:

♦ what is your moral stance

♦ what is your religious stance (if any)

♦ how far pregnant you are (the earlier the better for an abortion — before 12 weeks if possible)

♦ the nature of the relationship with your partner

♦ how old you are

♦ how far you have got on your course

♦ your financial situation

♦ your family's attitudes (though you may not want to tell them)

Whatever you decide, you may feel sad afterwards, which doesn't mean you've made the wrong decision. It's the nature of the decision itself: there is no absolute right or wrong.

▶ you may have believed that abortions are OK, but when it came to it, you may have found it hard to go through with it

▶ you may not have believed in abortion, but when it came to it, it seemed like the better option

To get an abortion ▸ you need to see a doctor, a GP, or someone at a charitable abortion clinic, for example, the Pregnancy Advisory Service, or a family planning doctor

▸ if the first doctor you see is unsympathetic, don't be made to feel guilty because someone else's views don't coincide with yours

▸ you can see another doctor or seek other advice (see above), and you need to do this without delay

▸ you'll then be referred to a second doctor — either at the hospital or as part of the abortion clinic set up

The legality

The ground rules are based on the 1967 Abortion Act, and an abortion can only be carried out for certain reasons, in an approved place, and with the agreement of two doctors who have to sign a legal form.

The commonest grounds for having an abortion are 'when continuing a pregnancy is more risky to the physical or mental health of the pregnant woman than if the pregnancy was terminated.'

Both being pregnant and having an abortion are very safe but, in statistical terms, an abortion is slightly safer than a pregnancy, so this leaves a lot of leeway for sympathetic doctors to help you.

❝ Both times I got pregnant I was on the pill, but had messed it up a bit. The first time I had *Jane is a 22-year-old student at Kent University* an abortion, I didn't really think about it, because I was only 16 and not that much emotionally involved. The second abortion was much more upsetting. I was in the middle of a really strong four-year relationship and very much in love with my boyfriend. I was two years into my degree, and really keen to finish, and I couldn't see how I could cope.

This time, it was a much more difficult decision to make. I was noticing changes in my body and I could feel something was developing inside me. This made my feelings about having an abortion much more confused and the guilt much greater. My boyfriend, although supportive, didn't realize how much it was upsetting me. He seemed to think that once the physical effects of the abortion had worn off, I would forget the whole thing. He only understood how I felt about it when he heard me describing the whole thing to his mother. Then he was much more sympathetic, **but I can still get very upset when I think about what I've done — even though I know it was the right thing.'**

Having an abortion

Unfortunately, whether you can obtain an NHS abortion locally or not depends on where you are living. Consult your local clinic or GP about this. If you need to consider a private abortion, expect to pay around £45 for the initial assessment, and then between £175 and £270 for an abortion less than 12 weeks from your last period (see below). If you have a 'late' abortion when you may need to stay overnight, then it's nearer £300.

Once you've been referred for an abortion, it usually involves more than one visit to the clinic or hospital. They rarely do it on your first visit there (which will be for assessment and discussion).

There are two main methods of early abortion. **Two methods** Which method you choose depends on how far pregnant you are and what facilities are available.

The suction, or vacuum aspiration, method:

- this is OK up to 12 weeks after your last period
- it usually involves having a general anaesthetic, which may make you feel lousy for a short while; but it can occasionally be done under local anaesthetic

- you don't have to stay the night; it doesn't involve any cutting; and it is very safe (but any operation has a tiny risk of something going wrong)

- once you've had the anaesthetic (general or local), a thin tube is put up through your vagina and through the opening in your cervix. It hoovers up what is inside your uterus and only takes a few minutes

The abortion pill — RU486:

- the advantage of this method is that it doesn't require an anaesthetic or any surgical procedure, and is therefore referred to as 'a non-surgical abortion'

- it only works until 63 days after the date of your last period (so needs sorting out quickly)

- it involves two or three visits to the clinic or hospital

- you take tablets (in the clinic or hospital) of a drug called RU486 or Mifepristone, which blocks the action of the hormone which makes the lining of the uterus hold on to the fertilized egg. The lining falls to pieces as in a natural miscarriage

- two days later, you go back to the clinic or hospital and have a prostaglandin pessary (tablet) inserted into your vagina, which helps your cervix relax and speeds things up

- you then stay at the clinic or hospital for a few hours until you've aborted, which usually involves strong period-like pains

- for a small number of people (5%), this method doesn't work and they have to go on to the vacuum method above

Both methods are very safe. There are few complications (infection being the commonest) and despite scare stories, long-term infertility is very rare.

Late abortion An abortion more than 12 weeks after your last period is best avoided. It is like a mini-labour: you're conscious and given various drugs to induce labour, along with sedation and pain-killers to help you get through it. So:

▶ be aware when your periods are due

▶ use a pregnancy test kit as soon as you are worried

▶ when you know you are pregnant, try to decide what you want to do quickly

▶ seek help fast

▶ if the professionals you are seeing are not being helpful, find another source of assistance quickly

Useful phone numbers

The Brook Advisory Centre: 071-708 1234
(they don't carry out abortions, but will give you a lot of basic information, and will tell you where to get an abortion if you want one)

The British Pregnancy Advisory Service: 0564 793225
(they have numerous branches and carry out abortions; you have to pay, but they are one of the cheapest options on the market)

British Agencies for Adoption and Fostering: 071-407 8800
(an umbrella organization for regional services for adopting and fostering babies)

food

You have to have it: you can't live without it. All you have to do is eat enough to stay alive. What you eat matters only marginally now, but it does have some long-term effects. 'Healthy' eating isn't to everyone's taste but it doesn't involve much extra time or money. Using skimmed milk, eating more bread, fish, pasta, rice, potatoes (all low in fat) and less butter, meat, and pies, is all that is required. Many of these things, as well as fruit and vegetables, are cheap and also high in fibre, which you need.

If you are overweight you are:

> ◆ eating too much

> ◆ not exercising enough

> ◆ both

You can eat in hall, cook yourself, or snack at will. Halls and college or university eating places are usually subsidized, so they are likely to be a bit cheaper than eating outside — or even cooking for yourself.

If you are trying to lose weight, eat less fat (as it contains more calories per gram than sugars and protein), stick to 'diet' drinks, and stay away from too much alcohol (high in calories).

Are you a nutritional disaster?

Try this quiz to find out how the amount of fat and fibre balance in your diet. For each question, put a tick against the answer which most applies to you.

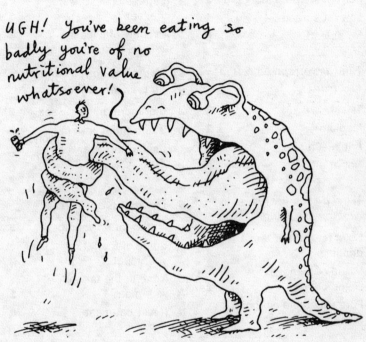

UGH! You've been eating so badly you're of no nutritional value whatsoever!

VINCE IS SAVED BY HIS POOR DIET.

SECTION A ★★★

1 *What type of milk do you usually drink?*

a Channel Island or gold top **3**
b Ordinary (silver or red top) **2**
c Semi-skimmed **1**
d Skimmed **⓪**
e Never drink milk **0**

2 *Do you use cream or evaporated milk?*

a Every day **3**
b Several times a week **2**
c About once a week **1**
d Less than once a week or never **⓪**

3 *What fat do you usually use as a spread?*

a Butter or hard margarine **3**

b Soft margarine **2**

c Polyunsaturated margarine **2**

d Low fat spread **1**

e No spread **(0)**

4 *How do you spread this fat on bread?*

a Thickly **3**

b Medium **2**

c A thin scrape **1**

d Not at all **(0)**

5 *What do you use for cooking or baking?*

a Solid fat (butter, lard, dripping) **3**

b Mixed or blended vegetable oil **2**

c Pure vegetable oil (corn, sunflower or olive) **(1)**

6 *How often do you eat chips?*

a 5 or more times a week **3**

b 2 to 4 times a week **2**

c Once a week **(1)**

d Very occasionally or never **0**

7 *What type of cheese do you eat most?*

a High fat: more than 25% fat (Parmesan, Cheddar, Danish Blue) **4**

b Medium fat: 10 to 25% (cheese spread, Edam, Camembert types and low fat hard cheeses) **3**

c Low fat: less than 10% fat (cottage cheese, curd cheese) **(1)**

d A variety of cheeses **3**

8 *How often do you eat high fat or medium fat cheeses?*

a 6 or more times a week **3**

b 3 to 5 times a week **2**

c Once or twice a week **(1)**

d Seldom or never **0**

9 *Do you usually eat?*

a All the fat on your meat **3**

b Some of the fat on your meat **2**

c None of the fat on your meat **(1)**

d Never eat meat **0**

10 *How often do you eat sausages/meat pies/burgers?*

a 6 or more times a week **3**

b 3 to 5 times a week **2**

c Once or twice a week **1**

d Seldom or never **(0)**

11 *How do you cook bacon or burgers?*

a Fry **3**

b Grill with added oil or fat **2**

c Grill without adding fat **1**

d Seldom or never eat these **0**

12 *How often do you eat savoury or sweet pies?*

a 6 or more times a week **3**

b 2 to 5 times a week **2**

c Once a week **1**

d Seldom or never **0**

13 *How many whole packets of potato crisps do you eat?*

a 6 or more a week **3**

b 3 to 5 a week **2**

c One or two a week **1**

d Seldom or never eat crisps **0**

14 *How often do you eat cream cakes?*

a 6 or more times a week **3**

b 3 to 5 times a week **2**

c Once or twice a week **1**

d Seldom or never **0**

15 *How many chocolate bars do you eat?*

a 6 or more a week **3**

b 3 to 5 a week **2**

c One or two a week **1**

d Seldom or never **0**

Now add up your total score so far

SECTION B ★★

16 *What kind of bread or chapattis do you usually eat?*

a Wholemeal **3**

b Brown **2**

c White **1**

d A mixture **2**

17 *How many rolls, chapattis or slices of bread do you eat on a typical day?*

a 6 or more **3**

b 3 to 5 **2**

c One or two **1**

d None **0**

18 *If you eat baked goods (such as pies, cakes, crumbles) are they made with wholemeal flour?*

a Never **0**

b Sometimes **1**

c Always **3**

19 *How often do you eat potatoes boiled, baked, or mashed?*

a 6 or more times a week **3**

b 3 to 5 times a week **2**

c Once or twice a week **1**

d Seldom or never **0**

20 *How often do you eat peas, beans or lentils?*

a   6 or more times a week   **3**

b   3 to 5 times a week   **(2)**

c   Once or twice a week   **1**

d   Seldom or never   **0**

21 *How often do you eat rice or pasta (spaghetti, noodles, etc.)?*

a   6 or more times a week   **3**

b   3 to 5 times a week   **2**

c   Once or twice a week   **(1)**

d   Seldom or never   **0**

22 *Which type of breakfast cereals do you eat?*

a   High fibre (Weetabix, Shredded Wheat, muesli, or bran)   **(4)**

b   Low fibre (Cornflakes, Rice Crispies, Start, or Special K)   **1**

c   A variety of high and low fibre   **2**

d   Never eat cereals   **0**

23 *How often do you eat a breakfast cereal?*

a   6 or more times a week   **(3)**

b   3 to 5 times a week   **2**

c   Once or twice a week   **1**

d   Seldom or never   **0**

24 *Which type of biscuit do you eat most of?*

a   Chocolate coated   **(0)**

b   Cream sandwich   **0**

c   Plain (such as rich tea)   **1**

d   Digestive, oatcake, wholemeal, crispbreads   **3**

25 *On how many days of the week do you have at least one piece of fruit?*

a   6 or more   **3**

b   3 to 5   **(2)**

c   Less than 3   **0**

26 *On how many days of the week do you have at least one portion of vegetables other than potatoes?*

a   6 or more   **3**

b   3 to 5   **(2)**

c   Less than 3   **0**

27 *How many cups/glasses of fluid do you drink each day?*

a   6 or more   **3**

b   3 to 5   **(2)**

c   Less than 3   **0**

Now add up your total score for this section | 20 |

SECTION A ★★★★★★★★★★★★★★★★★★★★★★★★★★★ **The truth**

| Less than 10 | Good! Your fat intake is low; obviously you have made some changes already |

| Between 10 and 25 | You are eating too much fat in your diet: you have plenty of scope for improvement |

| Over 25 | Yes, you are a disaster! Your fat intake is very high: it looks as though you really do need to make some changes |

COOKING TIPS:

A saucepan

SECTION B ★★★★★★★★★★★★★★★★★★★★★★★★★★★

| Over 25 | Good! You certainly know how to get your roughage |

A plate

| Between 10 and 25 | Your intake of dietary fibre is only moderate: there are some simple ways of increasing it |

A potato

| Less than 10 | Oh dear! Your diet is very low in fibre: you will have to work a bit to change things for the better |

A knife

Bridget from Swansea University

It's easy to fall into a rut of eating crap stuff which is more expensive. I sometimes make a surge of effort and go off to the farm shop to get fresh vegetables. This makes me feel really conscientious, but then they sit in the fridge going mouldy because it's easier to buy a ready-made stir-fry. The kitchen's a real mess and all the utensils are always dirty, so "cooking" anything other than bread, butter, and Marmite is a nightmare.

James from the University of York

I arrived here last October, nervously clutching a rucksack. Well, not strictly true. I also had three suitcases full of thermal undies, and boxes of emergency food supplies containing tins of dried potato in case of a potato shortage, and handy boil-in-the-tin chocolate puddings for any chocolate pudding shortages.

Emily from the University of East Anglia

The standard entertainment for a Friday night was (a) beer (b) a take-away (c) sitting and watching TV. When we felt richer, it was (a) more beer (b) a sit-down curry (c) going to bed because TV had finished.

My favourite take-away was chips and curry sauce, which I used to get from a Chinese restaurant. The proprietor always had me in stitches. Before wrapping the chips he used to say, "Sore finger?" It took me months of gazing at my hand and wondering which one he was referring to, before I realized he was actually asking, "Salt 'n vinegar?". Doner kebabs also went down well and if, on returning to the flat, I felt too full or too ill to finish them, I could always go to bed and microwave the rest for breakfast. Those half-eaten mermas and naan breads were delicious with cornflakes, and amazingly enough I only got very occasional attacks of the "two bob bits" after this kind of behaviour. I think I have evolved guts of stainless steel since becoming a student.

Tina from Cambridge University

'The great advantage of food in hall is that the meals are cooked for you; the disadvantage is that they consist of plates of carbohydrate stodge. There are no vitamins or minerals in the overcooked frozen vegetables, and no source of protein for vegetarians like myself. I am sure that this lack of a healthy diet contributed to the bouts of 'flu in college. The doctors prescribed antibiotics but never looked at why people were getting ill.

Friends of mine started missing meals, as they didn't like feeling bloated and ill. I missed one meal a day and took plenty of exercise to compensate for all the food I was eating. I fail to see how such unhealthy food can contribute to studying for a degree. **As the old saying goes, "Healthy body, healthy mind". Nobody at university seemed to have heard of it.'**

Bruce from Glasgow University

'When the college doctor asked me if I ate a healthy diet, I had to reply, "Well, I did till I came here!" At home I used to eat muesli for breakfast every morning. Here I eat two eggs, bacon, sausages, black pudding and fried bread, four pieces of toast with butter and marmalade — and all this after two bowls of porridge. This is because breakfast is part of the fixed charge that I pay the college for accommodation, and that way I can avoid spending any money on lunch. Dinner consists of more fried food, soggy overcooked vegetables, and steamed puddings with custard or cream.'

FAT   The average person needs to eat between 80 and 85 grams of fat each day. The table below gives you some idea of the fat content of a normal portion that you would eat at one meal (unless otherwise stated).

fat in grams

Dairy Products

half a pint of skimmed milk	0.5
half a pint of semi-skimmed milk	5
half a pint of full fat milk	11
a dollop of double cream	13
a carton of low fat yoghurt	0.3

Meat

2 sausages	21
pork chop fried with fat left on	25
pork chop grilled with fat removed	8
2 beefburgers: ordinary	18
2 beefburgers: low fat	9
roast chicken with skin	12
roast chicken without skin	4
fried streaky bacon	25
meat samosa	26

Fish

fried cod	9
steamed cod	1
3 fried fish fingers	11
3 grilled fish fingers	6

Potatoes and Rice

thin cut chips	17
thick cut chips	8
oven baked chips	7
small bag of ordinary crisps	9
small bag of low fat crisps	7
roast potatoes	8
baked potato (without butter)	0.1
fried rice	8
boiled rice	1

Cheese

Cheddar **19**

cottage cheese **2**

Fats and Oils

butter **8**

low fat spread **4**

olive oil **5**

Sweets

small bar of chocolate **15**

2 digestive biscuits **6**

The easiest ways of cutting down on the fat content of your diet are:

- try semi-skimmed or skimmed milk

- grill rather than fry foods

- stir fry vegetables because you need hardly any oil

- cut down on meat and increase vegetables and fruit (this is cheaper as well)

- use pure sunflower, soya, or olive oil rather than butter or

Most people in the UK are fat because they eat too much fat:

★ less than 30% of the total calories that you eat should come from fat

★ at the present time, on average, 42% of our calories comes from fat

★ fat has more calories in it per gram than other foods: one gram of fat contains 9 calories, one gram of carbohydrate contains 4 calories

cooking fat. Beware of bottles labelled 'vegetable oils'; they might be conning you that they are healthy when they are actually high in saturated fats

◆ eat unsaturated rather than saturated fats. Saturated fats increase the cholesterol in your blood and therefore the risk of heart disease later in life:

Unsats	Sats
sunflower oil	meats
olive oil	butter
soft margarine	full cream milk
nuts	cream
fish	eggs

◆ try eating more fish and fewer chips

◆ eat more pasta

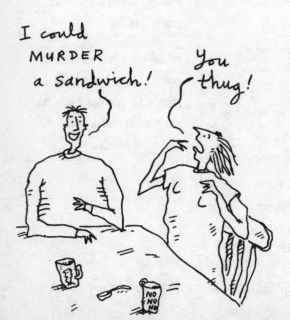

Proteins

◆ milk, cheese, chicken, fish, beans, and red meat are the protein foods which are needed to build your muscles

◆ you are unlikely to eat too much protein if you are taking in the correct amount of fat. Some high-protein foods are rich in fat as well (cheese, meats)

Carbohydrates (sugars and starches)

◆ they are cheap

◆ we need them for energy

◆ they contain a great many calories and not much else; but remember that fats contain even more calories per gram

◆ if you are trying to lose weight, use sugar substitutes in tea and coffee and on cereals, and drink 'diet' drinks

◆ bread, cereals, pasta, rice, and potatoes are all good because they are filling, are low in fat, and don't contain many calories

◆ many have a high fibre content (especially brown bread, rice, and pasta) which you need

◆ if you eat more carbohydrates and starches than you need, they will all get converted into fat

Vegetarian eating   • 14% of students (3 times as many women as men) are vegetarian, but many universities have not taken this on board in their provision of food

• you may still have to put up with eating the vegetables without the meat, or vegetables with cheese or an egg

• there is some evidence that 'fish eating' vegetarians are the healthiest

- iron is less well absorbed from vegetable foods than from meat foods, so eat foods with a high iron content like beans, lentils, chick-peas, eggs, nuts, cocoa, curry powder, wheatgerm, dried fruit, and green vegetables. You may need iron tablets which you can buy at the chemists

- the other vitamin that vegetarians may become short of (especially vegans who don't eat any animal products including milk and eggs) is B12. You will need to take a supplement like Barmene

- vegetarians should get their proteins from nuts, beans, lentils, chick-peas, rice, and peas (as well as milk, cheese, and eggs, if these are permitted)

Cheap tips (but not chips)

One large non-stick saucepan or frying pan and a wooden spoon are by far the best basic cooking utensils. Fresh vegetables, pasta, and fruit are cheap and good for you. Meat and fish are more expensive, but you don't need to have them every day (and if you are vegetarian, ever).

Recipe 1 ★

Stir-fry vegetables are an **extremely** easy, quick, and cheap meal — and anything else you want can be added. If you are feeling lazy, buy a packet of ready prepared 'stir fry' (two packets if you are hungry: frozen or unfrozen), and cook according to the instructions on the packet. Alternatively, buy carrots, broccoli, onions, bean sprouts, plus any other vegetable that takes your fancy; chop them up, and stir fry with vegetable or olive oil in a frying pan (you don't have to have a wok). Add salt and pepper and soya sauce to taste.

★ Recipe 2 ★

Recipe 1 may not be enough for many people, so boil some rice and serve the vegetables on top. Allow about half a cup of rice per person, cooked in one and a half cups of water for twenty minutes.

★ Recipe 3 ★

If you wish, add some meat, using chicken bits which are cheap. Cut into small pieces and fry in oil for about seven minutes longer than the vegetables.

★ Recipe 4 ★

Pasta comes in many forms — long spaghetti, flat tagliatelle, shells, hoops — the Italians have found almost every variety possible. It is very cheap in all its forms, including 'quick cook' versions, and all you have to do is boil it according to instructions on the package.

Produce a quick sauce to go on it:

- **buy one (there is a huge variety in jars, tins, and packets)**

- **or make your own to impress your friends.**

Pasta sauce

Cut up or grate one large onion and a clove of garlic. Fry gently in oil for about five minutes, then add a tin of chopped tomatoes, any other vegetables you fancy (perhaps courgettes), and some mixed herbs. **Cook for ten minutes while the pasta is on, and voila!**

You can fry some minced meat (a quarter of a pound per person) for fifteen minutes, and add to this to the sauce. A tin of tuna is an alternative.

Serve with cottage or grated cheese on the top.

★ Recipe 5 ★

A baked potato — one hour in the oven at Mark 6 (200 °C/400 °F) after pricking the skin — needs no culinary skills. It can be eaten with any of the sauces above, as well as with cheese and/or baked beans.

★ Puddings ★

Fruit and yoghurt are the cheapest, the easiest and the best.

★★★★★★★★★

CHAPTER 10

EXERCISE & SPORT

As physical fitness increases, research shows that:

▶ the ability to cope increases

▶ the ability to deal with stress increases

▶ depression decreases

▶ anxiety decreases

all of which is likely to improve your psychological well-being and your exam results.

The reason is thought to be that as you increase your exercise, you increase the beta-endorphins in your blood stream and it is these that help produce the feeling of well-being — even euphoria.

Mags from Newcastle University **'When I was at school, I played hockey, tennis, and netball, and competed in athletics meetings at national level** up until the age of 17. I enjoyed sport and still enjoy playing tennis, but what I didn't enjoy was the obsessive attitude that some people had towards sport.

When I got to university, I knew I didn't want to be in the "sporty" crowd. I did go swimming, and for a brief time got quite into aerobics, but only because it included a sauna afterwards! The most regular forms of exercise I took were cycling, going to lectures every day, and going out disco dancing an excessive amount. In the summer, I played tennis with friends on local courts. I like taking exercise but only in a disorganized and impromptu way. **The athletics unions fill me with horror.'**

Check your stamina

Find a reasonably flat route about a mile long (a bit of road, park, or running track). Walking, running, or doing a mixture of both, cover the mile as quickly as you can without becoming uncomfortably breathless, and note the time you have taken:

20 minutes or over ➟ **desperately unfit**

15 to 20 minutes ➟ **just unfit**

12 to 15 minutes ➟ **fairly fit**

10 to 12 minutes ➟ **fit**

10 minutes or under ➟ **very fit**

under 4 minutes ➟ **join your college team now**

Exercise

➤ try and find active ways of doing daily tasks (running upstairs, jogging instead of walking, bicycling rather than going by car or bus

➤ choose a form of exercise that you enjoy enough to do it regularly

➤ you need 20 to 30 minutes of exercise three times a week

➤ start gently and build up gradually

▶ you don't have to choose one form of exercise, try lots of
different ones

Dave from   ❝ I was a county tennis player and competed at Junior
Liverpool   Wimbledon. Now I play tennis, squash, and football. I
University   just about manage this along with consuming vast
amounts of beer, being fairly druggy, going out
frantically, and taking my academic career far too seriously. None of
these things interfere with one another very much. ❞

Types of exercise and what they are good for

Walking — great for stamina and relieving stress or tension, but not
so good for suppleness or strength; it's free, and an easy thing to do
on a day to day basis on campus

Swimming — if there is an ideal activity, it is swimming; it is brilliant
for stamina and suppleness, and for overcoming stiffness or sports
injuries; it doesn't cost much either

Cycling — great for stamina and leg strength, but not much good for
suppleness; a cheap and easy way to get around

Running or jogging — good for stamina but not so good for upper body
strength or suppleness; the only expense is buying running shoes,
and it is easy to do wherever you are

Tennis — good for stamina, suppleness, and leg strength; it is
possible to play all the year now that there are all-weather courts

Squash — you have to be fit to play, and if you are it is good for
stamina, leg strength, and suppleness

Team games — very good for stamina and strength; not bad for
suppleness, but to enjoy them you need to be fit

Weight training — with a suitable programme, you can firm up your
body, become slim and supple, and build up your stamina

Martial arts and judo — these involve a physical workout, relaxation, and skill learning; they are good for stamina, suppleness, and strength

Exercise classes, and aerobics — an all-over workout which is good for stamina, strength, and suppleness

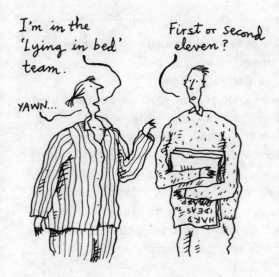

I'm in the 'Lying in bed' team.

YAWN...

First or second eleven?

Janine from
Newcastle University

‘ I haven't taken any exercise since I was fourteen. Cycling isn't an option as I can't ride a bike, so I walk to the university most days. If I could afford a taxi, I would certainly take one. In the summer, if the weather is OK, I do swim, but **I am dead against any form of organized exercise.** ’

Sports   There are two main types of sport: aerobic and anaerobic.

In aerobic sports you have to exert yourself steadily over an extended period of time, and this needs planning. Examples of aerobic exercise include: long-distance running, rowing, and swimming. These sports are good for conditioning your lungs and heart and keep you fit.

In anaerobic sports you give your all over a short period of time. The excitement is in testing your body to its absolute limit, but the sports do not in themselves keep you fit. Examples are squash and short-distance running. If you want to be good at anaerobic sports, you need to be fit. To be fit, you need to do aerobic sports. So if you want to be really good at squash, there is no point in just playing three hours of squash a day: you have to design an overall programme of fitness exercises.

There is also good evidence that keeping fit will significantly reduce the chances of getting a sports injury.

Getting fit

No single sport is going to keep you completely fit. Each sport concentrates on different muscles in the body, so to keep really fit you have to do several different kinds of sport. Most good athletes have a sport which they are really good at, and a whole range of other sports to keep themselves fit. Football, squash, golf, rugby, and cricket are not fitness sports in themselves, and people who want to play one of these sports well do other things to keep themselves fit.

Fitness sports include: running, swimming, aerobics, rowing, and weight lifting. Even these sports are not, by themselves individually, total fitness sports. If you are interested in being completely fit, you need to do a blend of sports which will exercise your arms, legs, breathing, and so on.

What is certainly true is that as you get older, training becomes increasingly important. Playing a weekend game of football will be infinitely more enjoyable and long lasting if you have done some regular fitness training during the week. If you don't train, your performance will be as great as ever for the first few minutes, followed by a rapid drop in performance, followed by wondering how you will manage to last until half time!

Overdoing it   It is possible to overdo sport. For instance, there is a great temptation in weight lifting to see just how much weight you can lift. This is not wise and is totally pointless. The experts in weight lifting do major lifts after long and careful preparation, including a rigorous training programme.

They know that it is multiple repetitions of light weights which build up fitness towards a single lift of the major weight. This may take weeks or months, and the same principle applies to any other sport. You may be tempted to go out there and show how far you can run, how fast you can row, or how hard you can play squash, but this is asking for an injury. What is infinitely better is to plan to build up your ability over a period of weeks, so that you can do that marathon, or row that six-mile race, feeling fit and prepared, and in the knowledge that you can do it without injury.

Injury means being out of the sport. It means that you have made the cardinal error and have misjudged your physical abilities.

Causes of sports injuries *There are three main causes:*

- playing when you're unfit
- poor refereeing (the game is not being played properly and fouls are occurring)
- incorrect use of equipment (the most common cause of injury in weight lifting).

It is worthwhile asking yourself, if you get injured, which of these factors played the major part.

Warming up

Most coaches think that it is very important to warm up before playing sport, to stretch your muscles and get the circulation going. It is certainly a reasonable test as to whether you are fit or not because if, after warming up, you feel you have used up enough energy to damage your performance in the game, you are probably too unfit to play!

The evidence that warming up helps to prevent sports injuries is still to come, and it is worth reflecting on the fact that wild animals don't warm up before hunting. In theory it seems like a good idea though.

How to handle a sports injury

The most common injuries are bumps, bruises, and sprains. As a rule, it is best not to play on with any significant injury because it will tend to make you protect yourself which will mean playing less well. There is also the danger of getting a second injury when your body is unable to guard itself adequately because the first injury has weakened its defences.

The first thing to do after an injury is to stop the swelling. The treatment for swelling is

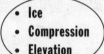

- **Ice**
- **Compression**
- **Elevation**

(remember the acronym 'ICE')
— the sooner the better and minutes count.

Ice — usually the most available ice is in the form of a packet of frozen vegetables (peas are best as they stay frozen for some time and can be moulded around the injured part).

Compression — is best provided by an elastic stocking or bandage.

Elevation — simply raise the affected limb above the level of your heart (with an injured ankle, for example, lie on a bed with your foot on some pillows, and wiggle your toes to improve your circulation to draw the fluid away from any swelling that is forming).

The uses and abuses of physiotherapy

Physiotherapy is widely used to treat sports injuries. Physiotherapists are especially skilled at suggesting a programme of exercises you can do yourself to bring you back to full fitness; and also at indicating how you can best avoid injury in the future. Never exercise an injury which is painful. Ultrasound, heat treatment, and massage may make you feel better, though scientific evidence for any other benefits is limited.

You are not fit to return to sport while an injured area is still swollen or painful; and going back before you are fully fit will leave you exposed to further injury. If you are off for more than a week, you will have to start a more general fitness exercise programme again.

Getting back to being fit after an injury

Interestingly, one of the first things that happens when you have to stop playing sport is that you become bad tempered and argumentative (yes, it happens even to top-level athletes). It appears that your body gets used to a certain amount of exercise each day and gets out of balance if it has a sudden change. So try and find some other form of physical activity which does not affect the injury and which you can do each day as a substitute for the sport which caused the injury. A rugby player, for instance, might swim or ride a bicycle. Once the injury has settled down, it is important to embark upon a graduated set of exercises to build up to playing the original sport again.

Overall, the message is: the sooner you get the swelling down, the sooner you can get back to training; and the sooner you start training, the sooner you will be fit to play the sport again.

' The great thing about being in university is the sport and the facilities. My school was crap at sport. I only had two games of football against another school the whole time I was in the sixth form. There were no tennis courts and no-one seemed interested. Now I do something most days — for the fun of it! **'**

CHAPTER 11

Blowing your mind?

On drugs illegal

Becoming a student doesn't mean that you automatically have to take out membership of the drug subculture either, but if you do join — whether wholeheartedly or occasionally — be prepared!

Ignoring the drug scene entirely is easy, perfectly OK, and often the preferred option. But if you are going to take drugs, even if you're just experimenting, get yourself well informed about their effects — both wanted and unwanted.

You may also want to be clued up about the legal aspects, and what your university rules are about drug-taking. Being a student doesn't put you outside the law, and some universities will automatically send you down if you are 'done' for drugs.

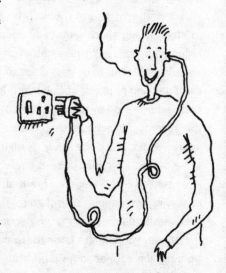

What mind?

Almost half of all students going up to university will have tried one sort of drug or another, at one time or another, but most studies show that students try a drug once or twice and then don't take it again.

No need for speed . . .

‘ Drugs, like most things, are available at university if you want them. My views *Roger from Huddersfield University*

on drugs have changed drastically over the past couple of years. I used to take a strong moral stand and thought drug–taking was completely wrong. The thought that people I knew might be smoking pot, or whatever, used to make me really depressed and paranoid. I just couldn't see the attraction; but I also thought there must be something wrong with me because I didn't want to take part myself.

Now, although I still don't use drugs, it doesn't bother me that other people do. I still wonder why they do it, because the idea of taking drugs doesn't remotely interest me. When it comes down to it, I don't want to feel out of control. But I can't tell people who do dabble in drugs to stop it, it's up to them, just as it's up to me to choose to leave them alone.

I don't feel any pressure to take drugs at university, and in fact most of the people I know don't take them. Those who do generally tend to gather in someone's room and "roll up" in there. It's not all upfront and out in the open. **’**

And that need for speed . . .

‘ It was around this time that I got involved with a group of people who bought *Susy from Sussex University*

and sold drugs. Not vast quantities, and they traded only among themselves and people they knew. I became part of a cliquy group of people, and in order to stay part of that group I needed money, as drugs cost money — lots of money. I also needed money to keep my new friends interested in me by looking fashionable, keeping up with the gossip, and having fun.

There was nothing illegal at first, and no one pushed me into it. Most of my friends were doing ecstasy, speed, and dope, and I could see that they were all OK. Nothing bad was ever happening to them. On the contrary, they could out-party, out-dance, and out-talk anyone else that I knew. I wanted to be like them — to be one of them.

I had fallen in love with this guy, who wasn't at the university and who sold speed, and anything else he could get his hands on. I knew it wouldn't come to anything, but me being the eternal optimist couldn't have cared less. I wanted to be with him all the time and my studies suffered.

Some of the first drugs I tried were "poppers"; they only cost six quid and gave me a quick head rush. I was in a night club at the time. It was excellent for about a minute: music and dancing were all there was in life. The next thing was I wanted to buy some ecstasy from my guy. I only wanted a third of a tablet, and he took the rest. I felt absolutely nothing, but apparently I was more talkative than usual and never left the dance floor all night.

After a whole tablet of "E", however, I became really paranoid, and this carried on for the whole day. I wasn't talking to anyone and eventually I ran away and couldn't stop crying. Next I tried some speed — only a half — and I loved it. I felt the blood pumping round my body: I could take on the whole world and be really creative. I stayed up all night listening to music. Speed is cheaper than ecstasy and more reliable, because with "E"s you're always in danger of buying duds.

By the end of that term I was hugely overdrawn. Then luckily I got involved with another group of friends who disapproved of drugs. At a party one night, I suddenly saw my old friends for what they really were. I realized that I had become bored with club life, and the benefits of speed seemed to pall. **'**

' **What I love about dope is the way it "throws" your mind.** It places it in a different frame. It seems to make your mind more creative, enables you to see life from a different perspective — to laugh at the mundane and not to worry about the present. Against that, however,

Mike from Edinburgh University

the long-term use of dope turns the creativity of the mind into sedation, producing slackness and apathy. Even when dope still inspires, it is all too soon forgotten the next morning. Indecision starts to replace action, and paranoia, reason. **I would smoke dope at a party, but not as a way of life.**

❛ Living on a campus university, and getting bored with the monotony of the Friday night disco at the Union, we decided to try something different. Seeking out some similar hedonists, our group planned an invasion of the local rave club. The entire week prior to this major event was spent organizing where to score the drugs and deciding in what quantities they would be taken. A mind, body, and soul experience was desired by us all.

Jess from Lancaster University

Rona, dressed to kill in her student rave attire, came skipping into my room. "How much are you taking?", she gabbled. "I've done half, but I think I might do the rest, as I've never done a whole one before and you have. What do you reckon?" "I don't know, woman, who does? But try just under one, and see how it goes."

In the living room of our flat, the music was blaring and the lads were having a smoke while waiting for the taxi to arrive.

Standing in a queue to enter the club, we all started coming up, with large inane grins spreading over our faces. Lighting up more fags, we started to dance. The club filled and our "E"s began kicking in fast. Gritting our teeth, fighting the rushes, we gave our bodies to the music. Nothing else mattered.

"Is Rona OK?", Tom asked me. "She seems to be losing it." Grasping Rona's sweaty hand, I slumped on a stool, unable myself to cope with the intensity of the rushes. "Do you want a fag? Do you want some water?" "I dunno what to do", she replied, grinning back at me.

In the toilets we locked ourselves in a cubicle. An hour later, or maybe longer, time had gone out of the window, we rejoined the hundreds of mindless dance machines, and idolized the music until the lights came up and we had to disembark. ❜

So how much do you know about drugs?

Try these questions

1 *The following is true of* ***cannabis:***

- it comes from the same hemp plant that is used to make ropes

  Yes/No

- it affects your short-term memory

  Yes/No

- it is the most commonly used illegal drug in the UK

  Yes/No

2 *The following is true of* ***ecstasy:***

- much of the ecstasy that you buy on the street at the moment contains no ecstasy at all

  Yes/No

- the effects begin in five to sixty minutes with mild rushes of feeling happy and relaxed and with no hallucinations

  Yes/No

- the relatively small number of deaths associated with its use have been mainly due to heat exhaustion and lack of adequate fluid intake

  Yes/No

3 *The effects of* ***LSD (acid)*** *last for:*

- 2 hours
- 4 hours
- 8 hours
- 12 hours

4 *The effects of* ***'snorted' cocaine*** *begin after:*

- 5 minutes
- 15 minutes
- 30 minutes
- 1 hour

5 ***Amphetamines*** *make you feel which of the following?*

- self-confident
- alert
- powerful
- energetic

6 *Which of the following are possible* ***side-effects of amphetamines?***

- damage to blood vessels
- muscle spasms
- fever
- serious psychiatric problems

7 *The maximum sentence for supplying or dealing in **cocaine** is life?*

Yes/No

8 *The following is true of 'crack'*

- it is usually smoked

- the effects start after five minutes
- the maximum effect is after ten minutes
- it is called 'crack' because of the popping sound it makes when heated

*The **answers** are in the information given below — see how well you scored.*

If you scored badly and you want to stay away from the stuff and therefore don't need to know, that is **absolutely fine.**

If, on the other hand, you are a user and you scored badly, **then you must be out of your mind.**

....

The facts and artefacts ...

Cannabis
Marijuana, blow, grass, weed, hash, pot, dope, shit, draw, wacky-backy, gear, puff

The legal scene: penalties up to a maximum of five years in prison for possession; and for supplying, an unlimited fine and up to fourteen years in prison.

The stuff: comes as (a) cannabis resin in browny-green blocks; the resin is scraped from the hemp plant (the same plant formerly used to make rope) (b) as marijuana: the leaves and flowers of the dried cannabis plant. It is probably the most commonly used illegal drug in the UK and is usually smoked in a joint or pipe, but can be eaten, or even brewed as a drink. 'Growing your own' is widespread. It sometimes contains other substances like 'horse tranquillizer', and fake puff is referred to as 'diesel'. It is occasionally (especially in the

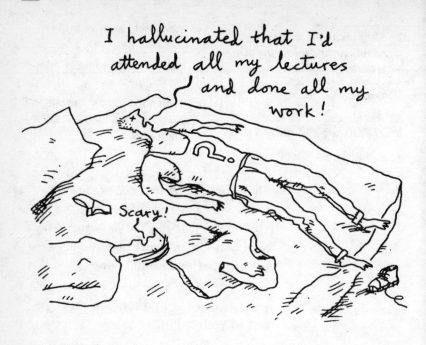

USA) adulterated with the toxic PCP (phencyclidine) which is a hallucinogenic. This can transform peer quality hash into something which has more effects than you counted on.

The good times: it makes you feel relaxed, it can make sex more fun, it makes your senses of taste, hearing, sight (colours, and so on) more acute, it's cheap, and the effects last several hours. You cannot overdose, it doesn't usually cause a hangover, and it doesn't produce physical dependence.

And the bad times: it reduces concentration and slows reflexes while you're smoking it; it can affect short-term memory; it can cause transient problems with vision; it can cause anxiety, and induces feelings of panic and paranoia. Very rarely it can cause acute confusion; combined with alcohol, it can induce a feeling of sickness. Long term it can have the same effects on your lungs as smoking tobacco, and it can make you apathetic. Though there is no evidence that it actually causes chronic psychotic disorders, the drug may modify the course of already established psychiatric illnesses, or tip someone into a psychotic episode if they have that tendency.

Specific damage limitation: includes buying from a reliable source, not taking it when you need to concentrate (when working, driving, playing sport), and not mixing it with alcohol.

Ecstasy
MDMA, E, ice, XTC

The legal scene: it is a class 'A' drug, incurring up to seven years for possession and life for supplying.

The stuff: comes in tablet or capsule form and is made artificially in the chemical form 3, 4 methylene-dioxymethamphetamine. The process of making it doesn't have to go all that far wrong to produce some rather nasty other things as well that are not good for your brain. Much of what is sold as ecstasy contains none of the stuff at all. Things like aspirin, barbiturates, speed, dog-worming pills, and a lot else besides have been flogged as ecstasy. Check out your source before coughing up the £10–15 per tablet or capsule — it's more dangerous than buying a second-hand car without an AA guarantee. Like LSD, whether the effects are good or bad rather depends on the mood of the taker before the taking.

The good times: if you manage to get any actual E, the effects can come on any time from 5 to 60 minutes, with mild rushes of feeling happy and relaxed and with no hallucinations. Heightened sensations and a feeling of exhilaration occur when going full blast in about 60 to 90 minutes. It makes you friendly, energetic, and generally delighted with your lot. The effects last up to 4 hours. Most frequently, E is used at parties to heighten the sensation of well-being, the sound of the music, and the energy to keep going. It tends to enhance the pleasure of sex rather than the desire for it.

And the bad times: some users get mild dizziness and nausea. The long-term effects are unknown (more worrying perhaps than knowing), but there are considerable concerns for both the liver and the brain — though damage may be due to the ecstasy not being made properly. Nineteen deaths due to taking ecstasy have been reported in the UK over the years, most of which were thought to be caused by heatstroke (in particular, loss of fluid as a result of sweating during active dancing and not drinking enough to keep up with this loss). Long-term effects may include moodiness, not being able to sleep, and occasionally paranoia. Ecstasy should not be taken if you are pregnant, or suffer from asthma, epilepsy, blood pressure problems, depression, or diabetes.

Specific damage limitation: a large amount of ecstasy is adulterated, so beware where you get it from. If you're raving, make sure you drink lots of fluids; don't overdose; and keep a friend around.

Amphetamines
Speed, uppers, sulphate, sulph, whizz, billy

The legal scene: penalties up to a maximum of five years in prison for possession; and for supplying, an unlimited fine and up to fourteen years in prison.

The stuff: it is made artificially and therefore frequently 'cut' with other substances, such as bicarbonate of soda and/or caster sugar. It is sniffed, swallowed, smoked, or injected — but injection is very risky because of not knowing what else is in the substance. Sniffing damages your nose, rubbing it into your gums can damage them so that your teeth fall out. The most frequent way of using speed is to swallow it direct or stir it into a hot drink. Effects come on within the first hour and last for about 4 hours.

The good times: you feel self-confident, alert, powerful, and energetic. It keeps you going for ages without food or sleep, but then

I've been noticing mood swings!

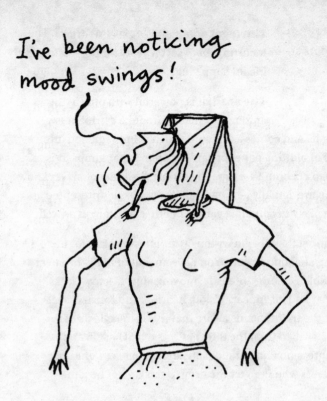

you collapse and have to catch up with both. When it was 'officially' available, it was used both for slimming and for keeping awake when revising for exams.

And the bad times: afterwards you feel tired and depressed, so the temptation to take more to 'keep going' is great. This can develop into very powerful cravings for the drug and the resulting high usage can cause damage to blood vessels, muscle spasms, fever, and very occasionally serious psychiatric problems including moodiness and paranoia.

Specific damage limitation: swallow, don't inject — almost none of the stuff is pure. Give your body and mind a rest after a dose.

LSD
(LYSERGIC ACID)
Acid

The legal scene: it is a class 'A' drug incurring up to seven years for possession and life for supplying.

The stuff: it is powerful with only a tiny amount needed to produce a 'trip'. It is artificially made, and comes as a liquid which is impregnated into small squares of blotting paper or card, or on to sugar lumps. It is relatively cheap at about £4 a trip. The problem is that you never know how much you are actually getting. Tablets or capsules presented as LSD are more likely to contain a variety of other substances as well.

The good times: these begin within 60 minutes and last for up to 8 hours, peaking at about 3 hours. You have an 'out of body' mystical sensation in which colours intensify, moving objects leave tracks, patterns appear and disappear. Vision, hearing, and touch are all distorted, but the user remains aware that this is the effects of the drug. No one has died from the direct effects of LSD itself; and prolonged depression and paranoia are known to occur only in previous sufferers who then try the drug. Users do not become dependent.

And the bad times: bad trips can induce acute anxiety, paranoia, anxiety, and fear; and at high doses, hallucinations. Don't take it if you are feeling depressed, and remember that the effects take a long time to wear off. Judgement and concentration are both impaired, which has resulted in the occasional fatal accident. It has also led to an occasional suicide. If you are going to try it, have a friend around to reassure you in case you start to panic.

Specific damage limitation: on no account take it if you already have some kind of psychiatric illness, and be prepared to do nothing else but cope with the drug effects for 12 to 24 hours afterwards. Make sure that you are in a 'protected' situation where the environment is calm and peaceful; and don't do anything that needs concentration, like driving.

Cocaine

Coke, snow, charlie

The legal scene: it is a class 'A' drug, incurring up to seven years for possession and life for supplying.

The stuff: it comes mainly from South America as an extract from the leaves of the coca plant. It arrives in the form of a white powder, cocaine hydrochloride, though the original coca leaves are sometimes available for chewing. The 'salts' form is often 'cut' with other substances which makes it very risky indeed to inject. Normally, users sniff it using a rolled-up piece of paper or banknote. Cocaine was part of the original Coca Cola concoction until 1903.

The good times: sensations of strength, omnipotence, and confidence. For these effects, it was used extensively in the USA in the mid-1980s by around thirty million middle-class Americans in social contexts. Initial reactions begin 15 minutes after 'snorting', but wear off in an hour or so. It doesn't usually induce hallucinations unless taken in large amounts. It is mid-priced at £50 per gram, which goes quite a long way; and at low doses has the reputation for improving sexual performance, delaying orgasm, and heightening sexual pleasure.

And the bad times: it can be very addictive and there is rapid tolerance, so you need larger and larger amounts to achieve the same effects. Regular use can induce feelings of depression, restlessness, weight loss, sickness, and paranoia. Repeated sniffing damages the membranes of the nose, but this and other effects wear off when you stop using it. Long-term use can damage the lungs and occasionally gives rise to serious psychiatric problems.

Specific damage limitation: includes knowing that whatever you're using is likely to be 'cut' with something else. Never inject it and be very careful about the dosage.

Crack

Freebase, base, rock, wash

The legal scene: it is a class 'A' drug, incurring up to seven years for possession and life for supplying.

The stuff: it is another form of cocaine, treated with chemicals to allow it to be more easily smoked. Smoking crack has a similar effect to injecting cocaine hydrochloride. It is called 'crack' because of the popping sound it makes when heated. Heating allows the drug rapid and easy access to your brain, causing an incredible initial rush, and unpleasant after-effects which lead to repeated use to keep these latter at bay.

The good times: the effects (not surprisingly the same as cocaine) come on after a few seconds and are at their height after 5 minutes. They include intense euphoria with a sense of improved mental and physical capacity.

And the bad times: the effects, at the maximum, last only 10 to 12 minutes and are followed by a feeling of depression. It is exceedingly addictive, especially for people who don't feel too good about themselves. Cocaine users who turn to crack get hooked on using it because of its immediate intense effects. This can lead to bingeing, which may continue until supplies run out. It has all the bad effects of cocaine, but more severely. It also causes enormous difficulty over sleeping. Frequent use may lead to hallucinations, suicidal feelings, paranoia, and epileptic-type fits. Regular users suffer from social and economic effects caused by the need to maintain supplies.

Specific damage limitation: this is a bummer of a drug that should not be used casually. Don't do it!

Heroin

Junk, H, smack, skag, gear, brown

The legal scene: it is a class 'A' drug, incurring up to seven years for possession and life for supplying.

The stuff: it is made from the opium poppy and starts as the opiate morphine, from which it is not difficult to produce the pure white powder of heroin — over twice as strong as morphine. Heroin is sniffed like cocaine or smoked. However, as with other drugs, injection increases the effects and is much more dangerous. It usually comes in very impure form: additives and infective agents are both present in 90% of street products.

The good times: with the right dose, you feel relaxed, happy, warm, drowsy, and content. There is little interference with sensation, co-ordination of movement, or your ability to think. At higher doses, you get an increasing sense of calmness and increasing drowsiness, until finally you relapse into unconsciousness.

And the bad times: after the loss of consciousness, your breathing packs up and you may die — particularly if you have taken other depressant drugs at the same time. Tolerance to the drug builds up fast so that higher and higher doses are needed for the same effect. Withdrawal from high doses results in 'flu-like symptoms which come on in 8 to 24 hours, with aches, sweating, chills, sneezing, tremors, and muscular spasms. Physical and mental dependence are both very difficult to avoid with repeated use; and it is very hard to give up.

Specific damage limitation: because it is sold illegally in impure forms, injecting is extremely hazardous. You have to know your supplier well (but even she or he may not know what's in it). Because tolerance builds up fast, leave lots of time between doses.

Overall damage limitation

- it is best not to use drugs at all
- if you do use them, eat or drink them; failing that smoke them. Don't inject them, because of AIDS, infections, and impurities

- if you do inject, always use clean needles (increasingly available from 'needle exchange' schemes)

- never drive on drugs, or do anything that needs keen judgement (such as mountain climbing)

- give your body time to recover, rest, and recharge

- eat normally and drink lots of fluids

- if you do take them, go somewhere quiet and safe

- if you find yourself getting caught in a drug scene you would rather not be part of, talk to someone you trust and try to find new friends

- remember: one of the worst things about drugs is that they are illegal. The police, a police record, getting sent away from university, going to prison, are not good for your health or your life

- read more about them: *Forbidden Drugs* by Phil Robson (Oxford University Press, 1994)

CHAPTER 12

STRESS & ANXIETY

Stress occurs when what life throws at you exceeds your ability to cope with it. The resulting feelings are those of anxiety.

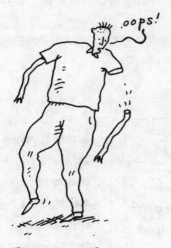

FEELING INSECURE

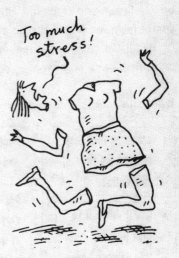

FALLING APART

What makes students stressed and anxious?

- difficulty in balancing work and leisure
- the demands of academic studies
- examinations
- difficulty in organizing work
- loneliness

- depression
- problems with personal relationships
- financial problems

Remember: whether you are willing to accept it or not, the truth is that **every single one** of those confident-looking, calm, collected students around you (which is the way **you look to them** even if you don't feel it) is as anxious as you are. If you don't believe it — ask them.

Students in all years suffer some stress; and although many of the main stresses can occur at any time, the main causes may change. In the first year it might be dealing with new surroundings and balancing work and leisure activities; in the second year it might be loneliness and problems with personal relationships; in the third year it might be financial problems and exams.

By far the commonest reason for students to seek help, though, is 'work-related' problems.

What students tend to do when work stressed:

- complain that they find it hard to concentrate

- find it difficult to take part in tutorials, and even miss tutorials and lectures

- complain of feeling tired all the time

- become passive and isolated

- begin to produce very strange pieces of work unrelated to the subject required and containing bizarre flights of fantasy

- become aggressive and start challenging anything that a tutor/supervisor suggests — even in the face of common sense

Some of this will be helped by work organization, which is dealt with in Chapter 13.

The results of stress

You will probably recognize these signs in those around you better than in yourself:

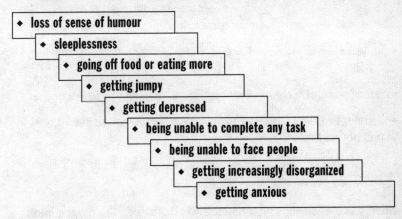

- loss of sense of humour
- sleeplessness
- going off food or eating more
- getting jumpy
- getting depressed
- being unable to complete any task
- being unable to face people
- getting increasingly disorganized
- getting anxious

These are not unlike some of the results of stress, but are more acute and include some of the following:

The results of anxiety

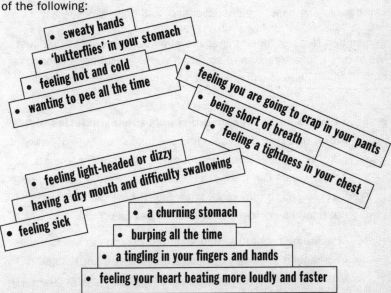

- sweaty hands
- 'butterflies' in your stomach
- feeling hot and cold
- wanting to pee all the time
- feeling you are going to crap in your pants
- being short of breath
- feeling a tightness in your chest
- feeling light-headed or dizzy
- having a dry mouth and difficulty swallowing
- feeling sick
- a churning stomach
- burping all the time
- a tingling in your fingers and hands
- feeling your heart beating more loudly and faster

So why do these feelings happen? When you feel anxious, more adrenalin from your adrenal glands (sitting on top of your kidneys) gets pumped around the body, which results in:

- an increase in the speed and strength of your heartbeat, making it pound

- an increase of tension in your muscles, making you feel tense

- a change in the blood flow to your skin and muscles, making you feel hot and cold

- increased sweating, a dry mouth, blurred vision, wanting to pee and crap, are all effects of adrenalin

When you feel anxious, you breathe harder to get more oxygen into your lungs and bloodstream which:

- makes you feel short of breath

- causes your chest muscles to tighten up

- produces dizziness, light-headedness, and tingling of the fingers

Remember: None of these things are at all dangerous. They are just the body's normal reaction to stress. If you drink coffee and/or coke, both of which contain caffeine, this will make these feelings worse.

Jane from Southampton University

❛ I could do so much more if only these anxieties didn't block me. How do people find the time to do "n + n" when if I did "n" alone it would be difficult? If I was more relaxed, people would like me more . . . but I don't really like people, I just pretend. If they really knew me, they would hate me . . . but I do like people, so why can't I just relax?

I'm letting my brother and sister down, and I'm wasting time. I do enough . . . and yet there are so many other things I'd like to do, but . . . So what? If what I am doing is good —

supposing my tutor thinks it is all crap? What sort of person would I be if I relaxed? Would I relate to people better?

I can't settle to anything now. I can't concentrate any more because of worrying about all the things I have to do. When am I going to do that essay for my next tutorial, when am I going to write those letters, when am I going to get that book read?'

Robin from the City of London University

'I'm trying to read Coleridge but I don't understand why one person opts for one subject and another for another? Also, what makes one person able to manage and another, like me, hopeless. I'm not sure why I'm studying English. It may not be the right subject for me because it involves me in so much work.

I seem to be up and down all the time, like last week I went to see the film *Peter's Friends*. I came out on a major high which blocked my anxieties for a while. Another thing I have problems with is friends. I want to make some really close friends with people at college, but in order to do this I must be in the right place at the right time.

My knowledge of myself conflicts desperately with the perception other people seem to have. Of course, my teacher is just being nice, which makes me feel doubly stupid that I am unable to handle any comment without dwelling on it and feeling uncomfortable.'

Should I be avoiding situations which make me anxious?

Managing your anxiety

You will obviously want to avoid dangerous situations, but anxiety can be a very real problem when it occurs in situations which are not dangerous. There are many things which are perfectly straightforward to do (walking into a crowded room, walking back to where you live at night, meeting new people), but which may cause you personally to become acutely anxious. Avoiding these situations may impose very severe limitations on your life, and in any case:

◆ you can't avoid them for ever

◆ every time you do avoid one, it makes it harder next time

◆ confidence has its own rewards: it is carefully built up by experience of being able to cope

◆ your confidence can be restored, however, by learning how to cope with small things and then gradually building up to bigger challenges

Is there a medicine that will make the anxiety go away?

Some medicines will help, but they are only a temporary solution, as medicines tend to work less and less well over time and some of them are addictive. It is therefore much more useful for you to learn some other method of controlling your feelings.

Nevertheless, although you will usually be able to handle stress and anxiety yourself, there are times when it is worth getting something like beta-blockers from your doctor. These will help in the short term. In the long term you need other coping strategies.

❛ **When it came to the week before my exams at the end of my first year, I folded.** I arrived home and told my dad I didn't want to stay at university, that I hated the place, and that what I really wanted to do was start right then making documentary films. We argued till three o'clock every morning. I've never seen my dad look so tired.

On about the fourth day, it suddenly came to us both that we'd been through all this over my 'A' levels. I just couldn't stand the stress of being judged by exams. Years of work, and you had to tell them all about it in three hours. Dad suggested seeing my doctor, which I did. It was too late for counselling, but she put me on beta-blockers and I took the exams and got a distinction.❜

I feel tired all the time. Can I give up trying to control these feelings? Will they go away after a rest?

Dealing with anxiety is itself stressful and does make you feel tired all the time. Not dealing with the problem now is just delaying things. Once you have learnt how to cope, the feelings of tiredness will go away.

Does this mean I'm mad and will have a nervous breakdown?

Absolutely not — being anxious means that you are normal, but you will have to learn how best to control this if it is interfering with your life.

❝ Well, I've got two more days to go till the exams. I've been a bit rocky since Friday, lots of tears and panics into the grey of 4 a.m. When I read my notes, they seem familiar, but when I ask myself, "What do you know about Diderot?", I immediately think, "Absolutely nothing." My mind is a complete blank.

I've been giving myself one day to look over each paper. It's not even enough time to read through my notes! When I started revising I wanted to cover everything. I've got so much material, and so much blood and sweat has gone into it all, but I just sit and stare at it and nothing happens. I can't go through life like this — I've got to find some tactics to be able to cope. Otherwise I'll feel a real failure. ❞

❛ Joe, one of my friends, just quietly disappeared one day and went home and had a nervous breakdown. He hadn't been doing much work. He maintained it was "all or nothing", and since he'd spent too much time on his "perfect" extended essay, he didn't have enough time to revise properly. So he lost all motivation to do anything. It's going to be even worse for him I reckon, coming back next year and going through all this again. ❜

' Sometimes I think, "Oh, it's not so bad. I'll do it somehow. I've always done it in the past." But these are rare moments! More often — like today — I panic. It's the last chance to look over anything, and so much of it seems unfamiliar. I have a horrid premonition of sitting down to the paper and not being able to write anything! The canon of French literature is so vast, and we do the work so quickly, that you don't have the security any more of going in there knowing they can't throw anything at you that you haven't done before . . . that was the beauty of school.**'**

How you can control your anxiety   *Simple relaxing routine*

Answer the following three questions:

1	**Do you sometimes feel physically tense?**
2	**Which part of your body feels most tense?**
3	**What makes you feel**

Now write down two or three situations in which you feel completely relaxed — such as sitting by a warm fire, wrapped up in bed in the morning, lying in the sunshine by a lake in summer.

You will need quiet surroundings, where you will not be disturbed, to practise relaxation, and you will need to practise a couple of times a day.

▶ **Lie on your back and take twelve very slow deep breaths, as deeply in and as deeply out as you can.**

▶ **Tense up for about five seconds as hard as you can, and then completely relax each part of your body bit by bit: your scalp, your face, your left arm, your left hand, your right arm, your right hand, and so on.**

▶ **Lie completely relaxed and think about one of the pleasant situations that you have written down.**

Repeat this three times.

Once you have learned to relax like this, you can use other methods to relax you when you are tense but can't lie on the floor!

◆ wherever you are when you get anxious, start controlling your breathing

◆ relax your shoulders and let them drop

◆ you will know by now which part of you gets most tense, so concentrate on relaxing it

◆ tell yourself in a controlled slow way 'Keep calm'

◆ ask yourself 'What do I need this anxiety for?' and 'What good is getting anxious doing me?'

◆ if you can't answer, tell yourself 'If it isn't doing me any good, then I won't bother to get anxious.'

Because, when one is anxious, it is difficult **Distractions** to concentrate on any one thing, it can be useful to go off and do something completely different for a time and come back to the problem with renewed energy:

> ‣ go and see a film

> ‣ go to a party and be sociable for a while

> ‣ go for a walk

> ‣ play sport or take another form of exercise

Panic attacks   These are very acute attacks of anxiety which can sometimes come on without there being an obvious logical cause. However, if you keep a careful record of what brings them on you may begin to recognize the kind of situations in which they occur. You can then work out ways of controlling an attack in these situations.

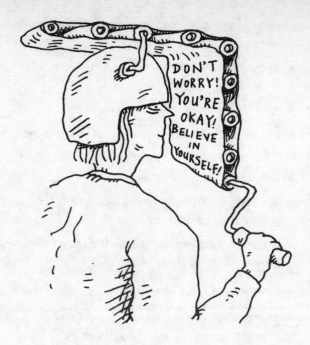

A PROTECTIVE HAT
designed to prevent
a panic attack.

Remember: You don't want to avoid such situations altogether as that will knock your confidence over being able to cope. Loss of confidence can be helped by facing your difficulties gradually.

Controlling a panic attack

When a panic attack occurs, it may be difficult to think clearly or to act sensibly. It is therefore a good idea to learn a routine beforehand of what to do when you have an attack.

- bear in mind that the feelings you get during an attack are normal feelings that everyone gets, and they are not harmful

◆ try and relax and accept what is happening to you

◆ don't run away; if you wait, the feelings of panic and fear will pass

◆ take deep breaths and try to slow your breathing down

◆ try and think of your situation in a positive way, giving yourself positive messages: 'Yes, I can manage this', 'I'm not running away', 'This is going to be all right.' This will help stop the cycle of more frightening thoughts coming into your head

◆ as you begin to calm down and feel better, decide slowly what you are going to do next to make the situation easier

◆ when the attack is over, think about which of the above actions helped you, and decide how you will use them next time

Record your panic attacks in a daily diary: what set them off, what happened, and what you achieved in overcoming them.

Recurring worrying thoughts

* I know I won't be able to write this exam

* If I go to this party, no one will talk to me

* I'll lose control of myself and be humiliated

* If I speak, something stupid will slip out and make me look like a fool

Overcoming worrying thoughts

The aim is to learn to recognize upsetting thoughts as soon as they occur and find some better way of dealing with them.

1 Write the thoughts down (no thought is too trivial if it causes you anxiety).

2 Read through the thoughts and ask yourself whether they are true (is it really true that you cannot cope with the next exam, go to a party, have someone to a meal?).

3 Write down the circumstances which set the thoughts off and ask yourself whether they have any use for you? Are you trying to protect yourself in advance 'in case' something happens?

4 Write down what you could do to stop that something from happening — a positive suggestion, like not arriving at the exam too early because waiting around with other people makes your panic worse.

5 Think positive thoughts to block out the negative ones — like planning your next holiday, or thinking about what you're going to eat for your next meal.

Insomnia

Not sleeping is often the result of stress or excitement.

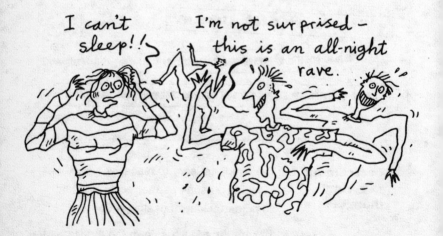

INSOMNIA CAN BE A PROBLEM.

❝ Lack of sleep so far has been the result of a hyperactive social life rather than from being overworked — although no doubt this is on its way. A lot of people cope with not sleeping by missing any lectures that occur before midday. In the long run, this is likely to cause high levels of stress, when you find yourself being thrown off your course because of not doing any work.

Jane from Homerton College, Cambridge

The beginning of term is quite stressful, because you're in a new environment and you haven't worked out how far you can push things like handing in work late, or being late for lectures. You're in a permanent state of tension in case you do something wrong by accident. As you grow used to it all, life becomes much less stressful and you find a routine to balance work and play. ❞

❝ Getting enough sleep is the problem at university, not "not getting to" sleep. Occasionally I can't sleep, no matter how physically exhausted I am. It's hard to be calm at these times and pass the time usefully — read a book, do some work — when you know that it is sleep you need and every hour is crucial.

Sammy from Bristol University

Sometimes I deal with it by taking a valium to knock myself out, so that I get a good ten hours and don't wake up as soon as it is light. My family doctor seems to understand this, but suggests that I shouldn't do it just before an exam, as valium leaves me with a hangover. As luck would have it, of course, the night before exams is precisely when I tend to be too nervous to sleep! ❞

Coping with insomnia

- lay off the coffee, tea, and coke which are all full of caffeine

- try having some other kind of hot drink instead (chocolate, herbal tea, blackcurrant juice)

- spend some time relaxing between finishing work and going to bed (different people need different amounts, but say, thirty minutes to an hour)

- have some exercise during the day

- read a novel or something relaxing in bed

- try tensing up your muscles and then relaxing (see above)

- listen to soothing music or relaxation tapes

- as a last resort, sleeping tablets will help break the 'cycle' of insomnia, but they are addictive if taken every night for more than about ten days

CHAPTER 13

An *easy help guide* to getting you through the work

Everyone works in different ways, and if you are convinced you cannot organize your work any better, don't read this chapter.

If, however, you do get somewhat hassled and think there is room for improvement; or if you want to try and understand some of the methods that are now available to help you work more efficiently (even if you decide not to use them) — read on.

❝ **I suppose my main worry about doing my first major essay was that I didn't know what my lecturer wanted exactly.** At university, you don't get the sort of individual attention you get at school (unless you make an appointment with your personal tutor), so you don't get the chance to talk the assignment through with anyone. Also, I'd taken a year off so I felt as if my brain had seized up through lack of use.

After much running around asking questions, in the end I just sat down, thought hard, and wrote my first essay in the way I best could. I know it's a cliché, but you can only learn from your mistakes. After all, as there'd been no guidance, how could they expect a perfect essay?

Oh, and a word of advice to anyone going through the "first essay syndrome": don't panic if you can't get hold of any research material. It's difficult for anyone to get hold of the books you are meant to use — particularly when two out of the three copies in the campus library are already out on loan. 9

6 Work was given to us almost instantly, I think one or two days after we arrived. It was mainly new work for me and revision for most other people, as I had only done single maths "A" level and they had done double. I found it totally hard, and thought I'd never catch up. As it happened, the differences disappeared after a few weeks. The rate of learning here is very intense. **We learnt the whole theory of "probability" in a term — something that had taken a year at "A" level, if not longer. 9**

6 My time is not as "divided" as it might be (into working or leisure time) as I spend a great deal of time feeling that I should be working but at the same time consciously descending into a state of vegetation. This entails doing absolutely anything to avoid sitting at my desk and organizing my life. Watching crap on daytime TV, playing endless games of gin rummy or Trivial Pursuit, chatting in our dining area, drinking cups of coffee, moaning guiltily about how much work I have to do — all these activities I have plunged myself into in order to forget about the mountain of books lying on my desk waiting to be read.

This doesn't mean that I find my course boring. Far from it, when I actually get down to it, I really get into the books I have to study. It's just that the actual process of shutting my door, sitting down at my desk all alone, and trying to ignore the sounds of merriment coming from the kitchen is tough, and tests your will-power to the extremes. '

'**The reading list was so long, that even if I had read from the moment I got up till the moment of going to bed, I would never have got through it,** let alone have had time for eating and drinking. Sometimes I think that the tutors who draw up the lists should try being students again for a few weeks and see how they get on. '

Work organization

Your reading lists may be impossible to get through in their entirety, so what are you going to do about it?

- take advice from other students as to which they think are the best books

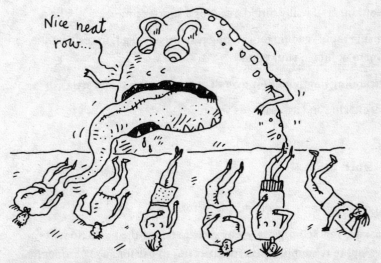

Nice neat row...

ORGANISING YOUR WORK

- listen for references to specific books on the list during lectures

- get a general feel for the books on the reading list by scanning their contents pages, as well as some of the text to see how easy it would be to get through

- limit the number of books you finally select

- if you can afford it, buy your own copies of the most important books so that you can highlight the text where you want to, and annotate the margins with notes (in pencil, so that you can change them if necessary)

You can improve your reading speed and what you learn from reading by:

- learning to 'scan', and trying to take in more words each time you move your eyes (best practised on novels, newspapers, and magazines)

- adapting the length of your reading periods to different kinds of material in order to maintain concentration (if fascinating, read for longer, if really turgid, read for a shorter time)

- using rapid reading for revising text already read, to reaffirm the main points in your mind

- scanning new books for overall content, interest and style

- criticizing and assessing as you read

Note-taking

Improve your note-taking during lectures by:

- asking yourself precisely why you are taking the notes (to write an essay? to remember facts for an exam? to use for an experiment?) and adapting them accordingly

- taking only selective notes (key points and key words to aid your memory)

- reviewing the notes soon after the lecture (if possible on the same day); this greatly helps retention of material

Improve your note-taking when reading by:

- reading the introductory and final paragraphs of a chapter, and scanning the subheadings, to get a feel for the overall content of a chapter

- reading section by section, and giving special attention to the first sentence of each, which may often be the key

- asking yourself (and answering in your own words) what the main points to be learnt from that section were

- making very brief notes based on these questions and answers in your own words (and not copying from the text unless you intend to quote)

Improve the quality of your note-taking by:

- remembering the notes are for yourself only and therefore should be pleasing and easy for you to look at and reread

- using a variety of coloured pens for different topics and to highlight points you think are important

- using abbreviations wherever possible

- varying arrangements on a page to suit the topic (diagrams, columns, spacing, underlining)

Timetable

Time management Work out what you are doing with your time by filling in a weekly timetable like the one below. See how much time you

	6–7	7–8	8–9	9–10	10–11	11–12	12–1pm	1–2	2–3	3–4
MONDAY	Sleep →	Up 7am / Breakfast →	Shower / Washing / To doctors	Lecture on George Elliot →	→	Lunch at bar			Chat with friend & shopping →	→
TUESDAY		Breakfast →	Work for 1½ hrs →	Break ←	Library / Finish essay →		→		Tutorial	
WEDNESDAY	Slept →	→	Up late / Missed first lecture	Had bath, washed hair / Listened to radio →		→	Lunch →	←		
THURSDAY		Up & washed / Breakfast ←	Read George Elliot →		Breakfast again →	←	Tried to do translation, went shopping instead			→
FRIDAY		Swimming with Gavin →	Breakfast →	Work crisis	4 cups of coffee	Quick walk	Phoned home / Went to get book from library →	←		
SATURDAY			Slept in till 10.30 →	→	Watched kids TV	Argued about where to have lunch	Pub ←			
SUNDAY				Slept in till 11.00	Breakfast & lunch ←				Linguistics	

are spending on going to lectures, reading, socializing, shopping, eating, sleeping, and so on.

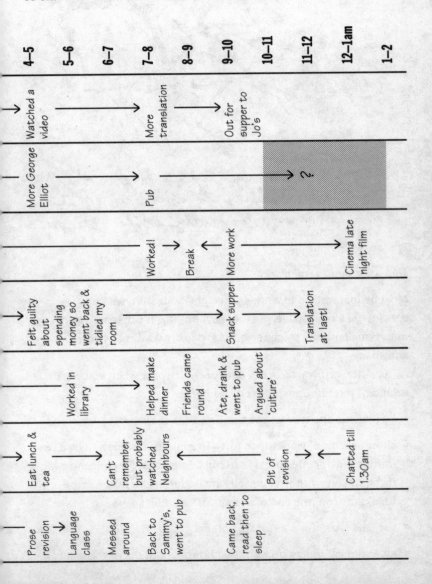

ATTENDING
LECTURES

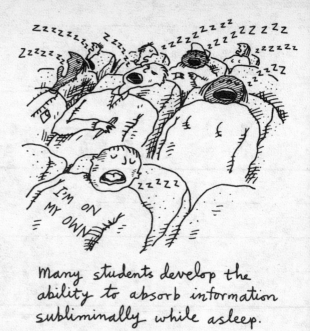

Many students develop the
ability to absorb information
subliminally while asleep.

How long should you work?

Most people who go to work do an eight-hour shift, which is
considered a reasonable working day. But this is broken up into
much smaller units by coffee breaks, pee breaks, lunch breaks,
and so on.

As a student, you have freedom of choice over when you work
each day, but this demands self-discipline.

- be realistic about what you think you can manage

- short periods of work (up to forty-five minutes), followed by a ten-
  minute tea or coffee break) are considered best for concentration;
  if you find even shorter periods are better, that's fine; natural
  breaks are too (the end of a chapter, finishing an essay)

- vary the type of work you are doing

- give yourself longer breaks spread throughout the day which can be in the form of rewards for work done — going to the cinema, chatting with friends, making love (this reward system works for any age and at any time!)

What are the best times for working?

You will have to find this out for yourself. We each have different biological clocks. Some students concentrate best at 7 a.m., others at 11 p.m. (this was written at 6 a.m.!). Do the most difficult work at a time when you know you work best, and give yourself treats (chocolate bars, apples, a favourite TV programme) for work achieved.

Where do you work best?

You decide. It may be the library, your room, a friend's room; or you may like to vary where you work.

Now draw up your own timetable and fill it in. Keep it flexible and 'trade' time between doing one thing or another. Carry the timetable around with you. It will not transform you into a perfect working machine (there is no such thing); but having a plan to follow will help in many ways.

It will allow you to identify free time to go off and do whatever you like. It will help to satisfy you that overall you are using your time efficiently. Most importantly, your life will be organized the way you want it.

Revising   It's no good being perfect in one area of study and no good in the rest if you are going to be examined on everything. So add up the total number of hours you have for revision. Divide this by the number of topics you have to revise, and allow roughly that amount of time for each.

If all the papers in the examination are given roughly the same amount of marks, 50% of the marks on each will be fairly easy to achieve and will get you through. Above 50% there is an exponential increase in the difficulty of getting a higher percentage. If you do brilliantly on one paper and get 75%, but fail the rest of them, you are going to be nowhere.

This is also true of individual questions on a paper. It is infinitely better to do adequately all the questions you are asked to than to do one question brilliantly but none of the others.

Some revision tips

- try to do some revision of your notes on the day you write them
- don't leave all your revision until three weeks before the examinations
- sort your notes out into subject areas
- make a daily revision timetable based on the weekly timetable shown above
- most students find it easier to revise one topic at a time rather than to leap about
- begin revising what you feel confident about, then move rapidly into areas you feel you know least about
- revise actively by summarizing your notes as you go along and use these summaries for your last-minute revision
- look at past papers so that you know the form and likely type of content of the paper, and do a bit of 'question spotting'
- keep making sure that you have time for relaxation and sport as these are essential and take away some of the stress
- be realistic and kind to yourself
- some people find revising with friends helpful
- everyone has different ways of revising — so find out what suits you best

❝During exam time, every exuberant, drunken, socializing cell of the university takes on a different shape — the shape of fear. This has become so common that exam pressure has become a standing joke. Everyone has their own horror story, and there are always willing and sympathetic listeners who have had it worse. Sharing stories eases the pressure as the listeners nod in understanding. Pre-exam traumas of hands trapped in revolving doors or emerging bloodied through broken panes of glass are always welcome. At least you know you've never been that desperate.❞

Examinations

❝Nobody likes exams. Everybody knows what it is like to feel your heart in your mouth, the need to rush to the toilet every five minutes, the panic of not being able to answer any of the questions on the paper. Some people cope with this better than others. However, I've done all mine now and I'm still here to tell the tale.❞

❝"Finals" worried me tremendously. They didn't represent just the finality of my degree, but the finality of my entire education from primary school, junior school, secondary school, through to university. This was it. Everything I'd worked for was going to be categorized by a numerical label, as if tattooed across my forehead, a scar for life.

So it all rested on a week of eight exams, and I was absolutely terrified. My heart beat so loudly at night that I couldn't sleep, and woke in the morning exhausted. I felt so overwhelmed by the volume of the work I had to cover, that timetabling was impossible. My thought processes became illogical and predominantly negative. How on earth can I revise everything and remember it all? What will happen if I can't answer anything?

I felt so guilty when taking time off, that "relaxation" was a contradiction in terms. Fear hindered my ability to think clearly.

Whenever I looked at a previous exam question I suffered mental blocks and panicked. Instead of treating the exams as an exercise to show what I knew about a subject, I could only focus on what I didn't know.

My goals were totally unrealistic. I found it hard to accept that I could cover only five pages in an hour as opposed to fifty. The perfectionist in me made it difficult to realize that you have to cut corners in revision, that you can't possibly cover everything. I thought only in black and white terms: if I couldn't answer a question brilliantly, I was going to fail. The fear of failure made my confidence and self-esteem plummet. Beta-blockers and sleeping pills helped to relieve the symptoms of panic, but they could not cure the cause.

Logically, my fears were unfounded. Examiners are on your side, they mark positively, not negatively, and they are not out to try and fail you, surely? **If I was going to fail, my tutors would have warned me long ago; and I would not have been accepted into this university if I was not capable of attaining a degree.** [9]

You all know the old maxim that some anxiety and stress before exams is a good thing as it gets your adrenalin going and increases your sharpness. The secret is not to get so anxious that it becomes disabling, so how do you control it?

If you know you go bananas before exams, and there is nothing that helps, it's worth seeing a counsellor, or a doctor. Some pills help, such as beta-blockers which definitely calm you down; but don't leave it till the day before the exams, as you have to get used to them. They can be a problem if you suffer from asthma, and they may, with some people, have other unwanted side-effects.

Some examination tips

- don't stay up revising the whole night before the exam; if you can't sleep, do something relaxing like having a hot bath

- on the day of the exam, keep to your normal routine as much as possible, like ensuring that you have your usual breakfast

- before leaving home, check that you have everything you need for the exam, that you are sure which exam you are going to, and where it is

- read the papers carefully, see how long you have for the whole exam, and spend roughly the same amount of time on each question (remembering that the initial marks on each paper are the easy ones)

- plan your answers before writing them, and if you are running out of time, use note form

- don't go in for immediate exam post-mortems: they'll be the death of you if you are anxious already

Remember finally:

- what you don't understand, you don't remember

- revising your notes on the day you make them is far more valuable for aiding memory than later revision

- getting some exercise (anything from making love to flogging yourself to death on the football field) is excellent for helping you to study

- keeping stress and anxiety under control is dealt with in Chapter 12

HARASSMENT

What is harassment?

6 **Harassment has something to do with the abuse of power.** It involves one person doing something to another person — exploiting them, or being violent towards them in some way, including rape — something which this other person doesn't want. 9

6 **As far as I know, neither myself nor my friends have had any experience of date rape or sexual harassment at university,** thankfully. I think the whole subject is clearer than it sounds. No does mean "No", and men are not animals incapable of controlling their sexual drive. 7

6 **I find it difficult to tell the difference between me flirting and me sexually harassing** — except that me flirting is appreciated and me harassing isn't. But how the hell am I to know how my behaviour is going down? 7

6 My personal opinion on sexual harassment — flashers and rapists — is that they are disgusting, dirty men, in desperate need of a shag. Either that or they get some sort of perverted high from frightening the wits out of, or ruining the lives of, innocent women. **I think they should be locked away and have their willies cut off.** 9

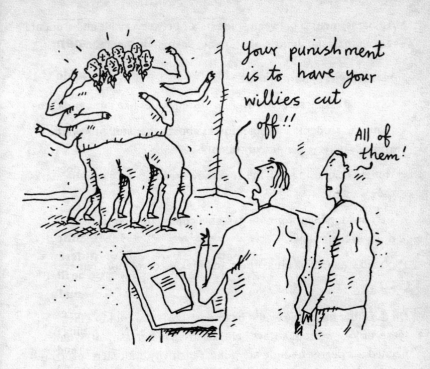

'Harassment is comments or touches or sexy looks that bother you. It can be teasing, gestures, remarks, or jokes; in fact, anything from somebody else that makes you feel uncomfortable about yourself or your body.**'**

'If you say no, that you don't want to have sex, and the person stops, there is no need to respect them more or trust them more — this is how it should be.**'**

'An erect penis does not necessarily need a second-party solution.**'**

'It seems to me that there are many things being referred to as rape nowadays which actually just need to be called bad sexual experiences.'

Most harassment is between students, or between locals and students — rather than staff harassing students or students harassing staff.

Some examples of harassment:

- locals harassing students over territorial issues like pubs and clubs
- groups of students making remarks about other students on the grounds of race, gender, or status
- students harassing staff because they haven't been given the marks they wanted
- staff making inappropriate personal comments about students' dress or their bodies
- pissed students pawing others and making derogatory remarks
- rape

On the other hand, life would be impossible if you couldn't flirt, tease, or joke without always being accused of harassment. What's needed is a degree of understanding, sensitivity, mutual respect, and common sense about other people's feelings.

❛ The second-years came down during Freshers' Week with roving eyes, on the hunt. They wanted to take their pick. They said really stupid things like, "Will you marry me?" They seemed to want to have a claim over the freshers, but they disappeared once it was obvious they weren't going to get it. ❜

❛ I first became aware of the situation at the end of my first term. One of my male tutors began to take an abnormal amount of interest in me. He was constantly singling me out for special treatment. Every day he would find an excuse to come and talk to me. Whenever it was time to have a coffee break, he would appear and offer me a cup. Although his ridiculous over-interest in me never took a physical form, I did feel very badgered. In a way, this made it more difficult. It was hard to explain to people why I felt harassed. They thought I was over-reacting.

In the end, I told him I didn't want to speak to him and refused to have any more tutorials. I thought he was going to be difficult about it, but instead he was incredibly limp. Afterwards, I found out he'd done the same thing to other girls. **❜**

❛ There are fights between locals and students, and though this is uncommon between girls, the blokes can and do get extremely violent. At some of the local clubs, the bouncers frisk blokes, and don't let them in until their pockets have been emptied and any offensive weapons surrendered. On some nights, students are discouraged from going there by enforcement of an "over 20s" policy.

The conflict is not only evident in pubs and clubs. In my university city, there are particular blackspots for students, one of which is unfortunately right outside the halls of residence complex. Within the first month, there were several fights between students and groups of locals. **❜**

❛ The only time I got hassled for being West Indian was at school. In fact, the only time I've ever got into fights was at middle and upper school back home. It's more subtle at university because people are more educated. The only thing with me was having a director of studies who quizzed me about odd things — like when I'd had a haircut, he'd say, "Oh yes, that's interesting, it means something special to you people, doesn't it?". Not exactly offensive, but just that somehow I was different. I stopped going to see him, though it was nothing overt.

John from Manchester University

I do sometimes notice in pubs and things that people are slower serving me and stuff. It's difficult to know whether it's just me being paranoid or not. I do know that Muslims and Indians in London sometimes get a harder time of it. *'*

' **I'd only been there a few days and was sitting having a drink** in the Students' Union bar. A boy I only knew to say hello to came up. If anything, he was more friendly with one of my friends. He'd obviously had a few to drink, seemed very interested in what I was saying, and stared at me a lot. All the time he was there — which wasn't very long — his hands moved further across my body, just wandering around. It wasn't threatening or frightening, just very annoying, and took me by surprise. I just said, "You've had a few too many", to try and make a joke of it.

If he'd been very big, I think I might have been frightened. As it was, the whole scenario made me feel uncomfortable. How do men have the nerve to put their hands all over a girl they hardly know at all? *'*

How should you deal with harassment?

In the first instance, harassment can often best be dealt with by the person who feels harassed. If you can, ask the harasser to stop by being direct and saying you feel harassed. Make it absolutely clear that you find the behaviour in question quite unacceptable.

If you can't manage this by yourself, find a friend who would be willing to be with you when you say it and will reinforce the message. If, however, you feel you can't cope with it on a face-to-face basis, write a letter to the harasser, stating what it is that you find unacceptable and requesting him or her to stop. Keep a dated copy of the letter if possible for future reference, should it be needed.

If none of this works, seek out someone in authority and get advice about what steps you should take next. Most universities and colleges will have an advisory panel, a counselling service, a telephone helpline, a rape crisis centre, or some other organization which will be able to help and advise.

Some tips

- keep a record of the behaviour that is troubling you, noting specific occasions of harassment and including the date, time, place, witnesses (if any), and what was said and done

- **do not blame yourself**; people often assume it is all their fault when it isn't

- malicious or frivolous complaints may be defamatory, even if they are taken to the proper authorities. They are likely to be judged as another form of harassment and dealt with accordingly

- many universities now have a written code of practice relating to harassment. If you think you have been harassed, you should get hold of it

What you can and cannot expect your college to do

You can expect them to:

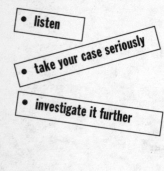

- listen
- take your case seriously
- investigate it further

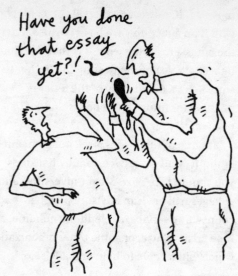

HARASSMENT

Given the complexity and subjectivity of these cases, however, it may be difficult for your college to take action. In some cases they can set in motion disciplinary procedures (these may be either college or university ones).

> But your college cannot be a court of law.
> It cannot act without objective evidence.

Confidentiality

Harassment and assault are extremely distressing to the victim. Colleges and universities are bound to deal with such matters in confidence. However, accusations of harassment or assault can, under some circumstances, also be grounds for legal action. Therefore complainants, those complained against, and the recipients of complaints all need to observe and to expect complete confidentiality.

Alcohol, its uses and . . . uses

. . . and seduction is one: but remember, if you 'consent' under the influence of alcohol, legally it is the same as consenting sober.

Yes, you know all the facts:

- you're more likely to have unprotected sexual intercourse if you're drunk

- you're four times more likely to have an accident on your bicycle or in your car if you've had alcohol

- each pint of beer contains 180 calories, so it's not good for slimming

- the accepted reasonable alcohol intake for an adult female is 14 units per week

- males, in this sexist world, can manage 21 units a week

- women have a higher fat and lower water content, and as alcohol gets evenly distributed in the water in your body, in men it gets more diluted

- some alcohol, particularly a little red wine, is good for preventing heart problems (but it is doubtful that the police would accept this as an excuse!)

- it takes about an hour to get rid of each unit you drink

- how quickly you feel the effects of alcohol depends on how much you drink, your sex, your age, and whether you have eaten

....

Some more facts: **Drinking and driving**

- the legal limit is 80mg of alcohol in 100mls of blood

- there is no sure way of knowing how much you can drink before reaching this limit — some will be 'had' after 3 units, some after 5, but driving ability is affected after 1 unit

- if you are below the limit, but driving dangerously, you can still be prosecuted

- young people are affected by drinking more than old people are

- one in five people killed in road accidents is over the limit

- if you're very drunk at night you may still be over the legal limit next morning, and no amount of showering or coffee drinking will get your alcohol level down (only time will!)

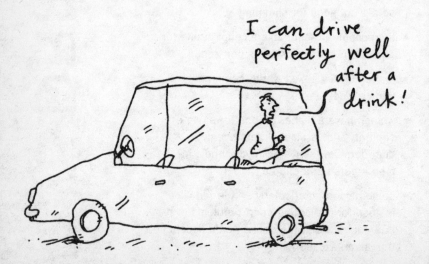

I can drive perfectly well after a drink!

Therefore:

- at midnight, after an evening's drinking, you will have 200mg of alcohol per 100mls of blood

- at 7.30 a.m., as you lie there with your hangover, your alcohol level is still at 130mg per 100mls (well over the driving limit)

- at midday, your level will be down to 80mg per 100mls (only just the legal limit for driving)

- at 8 p.m., not all the alcohol has gone, but it's OK to drive again

Just to check that you know:

one unit is equivalent to:

- **half a pint of beer**

- **a glass of wine**

- **a shot of spirits**

No, none of this will stop you from drinking — but it might make you think twice about how much.

Smoking   *Why some students smoke*

Mary from Chelsea Art School   '**I don't know why I do it, I just know that it's difficult to give up. It's a useful punctuation mark throughout the evening, especially in social or drinking situations —** definitely a prop. Films and television encourage me to see it as an addition to my persona, not just as a horrible addiction — which it is.'

George from Oxford Brookes University

'Everyone else did it at school, and I thought it would be cool. I know it's bad for me, but I don't feel it's doing me any harm — it just relaxes me in a tense situation.'

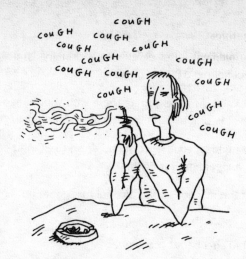

Emma from Edinburgh University

'I smoke because I like it, and it keeps me thin. Trying to give up makes me feel irritable and depressed. It's like a series of nice little treats throughout each day. I try not to think about the bad effects, though I do worry about them — especially as once in a while I get freaked by pains in my legs and arms.'

Why most students don't smoke

Anna from Sussex University

'Post-coital cigarettes really irritate me. I went out with a heavy smoker for quite a time, and smoke really bothers me now.'

John from Leicester University

'As I neither smoke nor drink, this certainly keeps the cost of socializing down, though in my first year it was a source of embarrassment and caused some social isolation. Nearly all the freshers' events involved "round the bar" camaraderie, and the feeling of exclusion, symbolized by a glass of orange juice, was often quite difficult to deal with. But I soon found a niche with a group of other non-smoking, secret lemonade drinkers, and we'd huddle in a corner, discussing the health risks of passive smoking.'

George from Manchester University

'Although I tend to thrust the health bit to the back of my mind, and I think the anti-smoking bit is overdone, I still can't see what's in smoking. It costs a real fortune, it smells horrible, and the girls I know hate it.'

What happens when you give up cigarettes

Within 20 minutes ➡ your blood pressure drops
your pulse rate drops to normal
the temperature of your hands and feet increases
to normal

After 8 hours ➡ the carbon-monoxide level in your blood drops to normal
the oxygen level in your blood increases to normal

After 24 hours ➡ the chances of having a heart attack decrease

After 48 hours ➡ your nerve ends start regrowing
your ability to smell and to taste things improves

After 72 hours ➡ your bronchial tubes begin to relax
your breathing becomes easier
your lung capacity increases

After 2 weeks to ➡ your circulation improves
3 months your lung functions are improved by 30%

After 1 to ➡ coughing, sinus congestion, tiredness, shortness of
9 months breath, all improve
the linings of your lungs regrow normally
your overall energy is improved

After 5 years ➡ lung cancer death risk for the average smoker
decreases from 137 per 100,000 people to 72,
and after 10 years to 12 (which is almost the rate
for non-smokers)

After 10 years ➡ all pre-cancerous cells have been replaced
other cancers, such as those of the mouth, throat,
bladder, kidney and cervix, are decreased as well

Some things to help you:

If you do smoke and are trying to give up

- first you have to want to give up

- pick a day and then take each day at a time

- be aware of situations when you normally must have a cigarette (at parties, when drinking, or when studying late at night: these are 'danger spots' and you need to work out how you are going to deal with them)

- make a pact with a friend who is a smoker and also wants to give up

- avoid friends who smoke and tend to push you to have one (in order to make themselves feel better)

- don't worry about gaining weight — you will lose it again

- try to have your first cigarette as late in the day as possible

- take pride in the fact that you will be decreasing the profits of tobacco companies and their contributions to other organizations you might not want to support

- treat yourself to something you really want with the money you have saved

- each time you have a cigarette, make yourself give a donation to the National Front

Other things that might help are nicotine chewing gum or patches. They are not available on prescription but they are cheaper than the cigarettes you would be smoking. It often helps to use these, and at the same time see your doctor or nurse because then there's someone else that you will find difficult to let down.

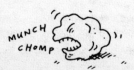

CHAPTER 16

When you've got *body rot*

Your body won't behave itself the way you want it to all the time. It will ache, get feverish, come out in spots, tell you that it doesn't want to go on . . . It will get invaded by the odd virus or bacteria. Most of these attacks will get better on their own, but some will need the attention of a doctor.

Your body will also need a bit of tender, loving care, the odd morsel of food, and occasional abstinence from sex, drugs, and alcohol — if that's what made it out of sorts.

It is worth noting that a couple of days of 'flu or some other illness will not be regarded as an excuse, by the powers that be, for having done no work at all for a whole term. If you do have an illness which is affecting your work, you should have no difficulty in getting a medical certificate, and your college is likely to be sympathetic.

Aspirin or paracetamol will help most things, and three-quarters of students appear to have these among their belongings. Doctors won't be very sympathetic if you call them out just for aspirin or paracetamol!

As an insurance policy, it's a good idea to be sympathetic and helpful to those around you who get ill, so that in your hour of need, someone is sympathetic and helpful in return...

Kate from Cambridge University

❛ There is great pressure on you not to get ill. Even though the life-style led by students tends to run you down, you somehow keep going until the end of term, ignoring any symptoms, and then collapse as soon as you get home.

However, I did not manage to ignore the acute attack of 'flu I got just before my major medical exams this year. Because of the timing, I was made to feel I was pretending, and that all it was was pre-exam panic. Normally, I actually work best under pressure and feel very clear-headed just before exams. This particular day I felt sweaty and exhausted; the more I tried to revise, the thicker my head felt and the foggier everything became. I battled on, and as I realized nothing was going in, I began to get mildly hysterical. The combination of fever, tiredness, and panic sent me into fits of crying which made everything worse.

In the end, I telephoned my doctor, having been made to feel a fake by my house-mates, who sat around downstairs reading through their notes and looking mildly bemused by my screaming confusion. The doctor was very nice. By the time he came, I had slept a lot of it off, taken aspirin, and felt generally much better. He offered to write me a note for the next day's exam, and said I should ring if I felt worse in the morning. Luckily I woke up feeling a great deal better, just snotty and with slightly swollen glands. The exam went OK, so I didn't bother to get that note.

Although it was nothing serious, I felt I didn't have a minute to waste by being ill. I'm not an attention seeker, and it was awful to feel as though I must be pretending.[9]

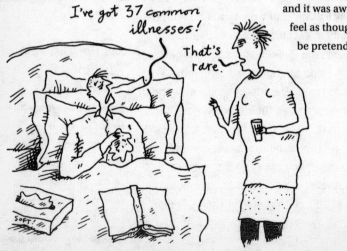

These are extremely common, and will become familiar friends at university. They often come together and are easily caught from other people when living in close proximity.

Coughs and colds

They are usually caused by: viruses, which are not killed off by antibiotics, so are best dealt with on your own. Doctors and nurses have no magic cures; nor do the drug companies peddling expensive 'cold cures' and 'cough mixtures'.

The best treatment is: aspirin or paracetamol (the cheapest are the best), warm drinks, being nice to yourself, and patience — all of which will, in the long run, make you feel better. Sympathy from someone else is also wonderful, so build up a few Brownie points with others suffering from coughs and colds. Inhalations and decongestants, such as Sudafed, will sometimes make you feel more clear-headed but won't speed up recovery.

They usually last: at least a week.

You need to see a doctor:

▶ if coughing continues a week or two after a cold has cleared up
▶ if coughing produces dirty yellow or green phlegm
▶ if you cough up blood
▶ if you get short of breath
▶ if you have a high fever (39.5 °C or above) which continues
▶ if you feel worried about yourself

Sore throats   These are also very common and can get quite nasty. You often get swelling in the glands in your neck, as well as a sore throat, and these become painful too. This is the body's normal way of dealing with infection.

They are mainly (65%) caused by: viruses which antibiotics cannot cure. Sometimes they are caused by a bacteria (this is usually called a 'strep throat'). It is difficult to tell the difference between a viral or a bacterial sore throat, but taking an antibiotic doesn't normally affect how long you're ill. If you look down your throat in the mirror, and your tonsils are covered with white spots, it's probably worth seeing your doctor for some antibiotics.

The best treatment is: gargling with 2 soluble aspirin in water every 4 hours and then swallowing, as this will usually ease the pain and make you feel better. You may not feel like eating much, so just keep drinking plenty of fluids.

They usually last: 4 to 5 days.

You need to see your doctor:

▸ if the sore throat is still getting worse after 2 days
▸ if you have bad earache as well
▸ if you have a high temperature which doesn't go down (over 39.5 °C)
▸ if you can't swallow at all

Most sore throats are not glandular fever (though glandular fever often starts with a sore throat).

Diarrhoea and vomiting (D and V)

This is another ailment you might get. At worst, you may have both problems together but they frequently happen independently, at one end or the other. You may get some tummy cramps with D and V. If you've just got back from exotic foreign parts and have D and V or develop it, see your doctor.

It is usually caused by: viruses which you catch from other people, but occasionally because some food you've eaten has got infected by a bug, or hasn't been cooked properly. If this is the case, you'll find you're not alone in the lavatory as whole halls of residence may get D and V at the same time.

The best treatment is: stopping eating (which you probably won't feel like, and you won't waste away over a few days). Carry on drinking fluids, frequently, in small amounts. Fizzy water, coke, and lemonade are all fine. Milky drinks are best avoided. When you start to feel better, gradually begin eating again, but avoid large and fatty meals.

Normally D and V begin to settle: after 48 hours.

You may need to see the doctor:

▶ **if the diarrhoea doesn't start to get better after 48 hours**

▶ **if the vomiting goes on for more than 24 hours**

▶ **if you begin to get a lot of tummy pain**

▶ **if there is blood or mucus in your diarrhoea**

▶ **if you've just returned from overseas**

This is a lousy trick played by nature, just as you're about to take your examinations, go to the best party of your life, or begin your holidays.   **FLU**

⁶ **Within the first two weeks of my first term, everyone — and I mean everyone — was ill.** I came down with "fresher's flu" and had to spend three days in bed. I was worried that no one would notice my absence from the social scene or that I'd get stern notes of warning about missing lectures. But thankfully a couple of friends popped in to see me between tutorials, and the warden's wife brought me gallons of orange juice to slurp down. I was also seen by the campus doctor, who nodded sympathetically as I croaked away. So, despite hardly being able to breathe, having flu away from home wasn't too grim an experience. In fact, I was more worried about sniffing and coughing on the phone to Mum and Dad, who are the world's biggest worriers.⁹

Real flu is caused by: one of the influenza viruses, of which there are a multitude (Hong Kong, Asian, Red; notice that they are always caused by foreigners: the British are never to blame!).

However, there is a huge range of other nasty little buggers which cause flu-like problems. You feel lousy, get a fever, ache all over, have a bit of a sore throat and a slightly runny nose, and you want to curl up (without anybody else) in bed.

The best treatment is: aspirin or paracetamol and lots to drink. Go to bed if you feel like it, and you probably will. Find someone sympathetic, and get a friend to tell your tutor why you haven't done the work you should have. Most important: stay away from the doctor so that she or he doesn't get it!

Spots

Danny from Durham University

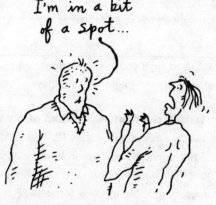

I'm in a bit of a spot...

⁶**I wake up on a sunny day in Durham.** It's the first term of my first year at university and I feel good. The opportunities being presented to me now are greater than those I have ever had before. New friends, new interests . . . and new spots.

New spots force me into subterfuge. Instinctively, the first thing I do upon waking — before even getting out of bed — is feel my chin, nose, and forehead. I'm checking for any new eruptions of pus that have appeared during the night. I find bumps. Three in total. But my fingers also detect something much worse — a white-headed spot. It just isn't fashionable — not now, not ever. I must squeeze that spot.

SPLAT. It's over in seconds. But unfortunately I squeeze too hard and the crater which, only a few moments ago, was filled with pus, is now filled with blood. I hear voices coming down the corridor. My neighbours are awake. I'm not fit to enter the social scene.⁹

Treatment helps: and most of you who have still got acne now will have tried over-the-counter stuff. There are remedies which doctors can offer in the way of stronger lotions and potions and antibiotics, so it is worth going to consult one, who will (or should) be helpful and sympathetic.

Headaches

These are extremely common and can be caused by a variety of things — stress, anxiety, and tension being the commonest. Headaches are also usual with any fever. Most of them will settle with relaxation, exercise, or a few aspirin or paracetamol.

Of course, what students actually worry about is whether they have brain cancer or meningitis. OK — so for every million or so headaches, there will be one case of one of these. So if you do have a very severe headache, associated with feeling very ill and having a very high fever, or if you have a headache which doesn't go away, or your neck feels stiff — see your doctor immediately.

Glandular fever

This is caused by: the Epstein Barr virus, called after the men who first described it. It is very common, and by the age of 18 many of you will have had it already — some without even knowing. It spreads from one person to another by close contact, which is why it's known as the 'kissing' disease; but kissing isn't the only way of getting it. It can be spread by breathing the virus in, or swallowing it.

The symptoms you will notice are: that your throat is sore, and that you have swollen glands in your neck, and sometimes under your arms, or in your groin. You may also feel tired and unwell, have a headache, a fever, and occasionally a rash. The doctor can do a blood test to prove that you've got it (or that you've had it in the past) but it doesn't always show up positive immediately. There are other diseases which make you feel the same way, but these don't give a positive glandular fever test.

Treatment is: mainly looking after yourself. There isn't anything special that doctors can give you (though your doctor may already have given you antibiotics for your sore throat before it was diagnosed as glandular fever). If you get very swollen glands, a short course of steroids may help to decrease the swelling. Mostly, it is up to you to take aspirin or paracetamol to help bring your fever down, help the pain in your throat, and generally make you feel better. How much activity you undertake, and whether you take to your bed or not, depends on how ill you feel. If you know you've got it, it's best not do sports or drink alcohol during the first 3 weeks of the illness, but you probably won't feel like either. Be guided by how you feel.

It usually lasts: about 3 weeks. In the first week, you have a sore throat, swollen glands, and fever, and probably feel like staying in bed. In the second week, you feel a bit better but still pretty tired. In the third week, you will probably still feel tired and not like doing too much. A tiny minority feel tired for weeks or months afterwards (see below).

You should see your doctor:

- **if you have a sore throat, enlarged glands, and tiredness and fever which doesn't clear up within 3 days (though most of these will not be glandular fever!)**
- **if you feel really tired and unwell, and still have a bit of fever after a sore throat has gone away**

Feeling tired all the time   This is an extremely common problem among students. There are many different possible reasons, such as too many late-night parties, or over-indulgence in sex, drugs, and alcohol. Under-indulgence in these can also give rise to the same problem because you feel lonely, isolated, and depressed — all good reasons for feeling tired

all the time. These problems are dealt with in Chapter 18.
Illnesses caused by viruses and bacteria are likely to have the same effect, and most of these you get over quickly. However, there is a group of rather vague illnesses which can cause tiredness but are not easy to define.

Fiona from St. Andrews University

' I just felt totally and utterly exhausted all the time, whatever I did. It was as if every cell in my body had run out of energy. I don't know how they all held together. I walked, talked, worked, ate, slept in a state of continually thinking, "I can't go on, I can't do another thing. I'm at my last gasp. Why struggle all the time?" And yet I did go on: dragging myself reluctantly here and there, like some pathetic, washed-out rag, until at last I couldn't stand it any longer and went to see my tutor.

She sent me to my doctor, who sent me on to the university counsellor, to whom I tearfully admitted how I was feeling — behind with all my work, my essays not up to scratch, and not sleeping at night. The instant revelation was that I wasn't suffering from some terrible disease. This is what had been really causing me angst, and it took me a long time to get over it. At least it got me thinking about what I was trying to do, got me to organize myself a little, work out some priorities, and basically just took the immediate strain away.'

Paul from the University of East London

' After an enjoyable one and a bit years at university, I suddenly developed a 'flu-like illness: a disabling fatigue and a total inability to concentrate. After some medical investigations (all negative), I was advised that I was "just" suffering from a virus, and to carry on with my studies. Trusting in the doctors, I followed their advice — advice that was repeated over the next few months as I struggled on with wildly fluctuating symptoms. A year later I suffered a complete relapse.

I was given leave of absence and returned home virtually bed-bound. An interested GP referred me to a specialist, who promptly diagnosed ME (Myalgic Encephalitis). Until recently, I thought I was a unique phenomenon but I have been shocked to find that this is not so.[9]

Chronic Fatigue Syndrome or Myalgic Encephalitis (ME, post-viral syndrome, yuppy flu)

Myalgic Encephalitis is a medical term which in translation means 'pain in the muscles and inflammation of the brain'.

There is controversy and scepticism as to the existence and exact nature of ME. People do get lethargic, tired, and lacking in energy after a viral illness like glandular fever or flu. In a few people, these problems can go on for many months, or longer.

The specific symptoms of ME include:

- **aching in the muscles after exercise**
- **memory loss**
- **difficulty in concentrating**
- **depression**

after a non-specific viral illness, or apparently 'out of the blue'. Nobody knows why it affects some people and not others; and what makes matters more difficult is that, up to the present time, there is no specific test which tells you whether you have chronic fatigue syndrome or not.

More and more people are now convinced that it does exist, but nobody knows how to treat it effectively. Rest, anti-depressants, alternative medicines, and a gradual exercise programme, have all been tried with varying degrees of success. However, it does appear to get better by itself, even if it takes some time, and it remains a not uncommon reason for students having to take time off university. Only a minority of people go on to have persistent problems with it. If you think you have got it contact your doctor.

CHAPTER

Parts rot

sexually transmitted diseases

> Warning: reading this may put you off sex, OR
> it may save your sex life for ever

'After about ten minutes of general conversation and some kettle, teabag and mug co-ordination, Simon suddenly decided to "hit me" with his genital warts. This was completely unsolicited and prompted by nothing we'd been talking about. I'm not unsympathetic to Simon and his problems (he has, after all, got enough — believe me), but if I want to hear this kind of thing out of the blue, I tend, for preference, to watch Oprah Winfrey. In any case, I wanted to go out. But this is how it happened.

Chrissy from Glasgow University

Simon suddenly said, "God I'm knackered, I had to be at Clinic 1A at six-thirty this morning." Having a vague suspicion of what Clinic 1A entailed, I just said, "Oh really? Isn't that where you go if you have some kind of sexually transmitted disease?" "Exactly," he went on. I thought he might. "I went to get my genital warts treated. I've had them for ages, because when I got home I didn't get them treated properly and they grew back again."

Not having anything of my own along these lines to share, I just said, "Oh", and asked him if he'd told his parents. "I've told my mum. She didn't say much." "Great," I thought, "end of conversation." I wouldn't have to find out what they look like or who had given them to him.

"They're not painful or anything. I got them off my ex–girlfriend, Sylvia." Oh no, here comes the whole story. "Yes, she slept with some waiter she met in Cyprus." He stopped, and then added, "A bit slaggy, I suppose, and she didn't know she had them until she'd given them to me. At the time, I was so obsessed with her I just said I didn't mind."

Talk about loving someone warts and all . . . I think I might have said something a lot worse! After he left, I felt as if I'd participated in one of those "true confession" shows, where you stand up and say, "Hello, my name is Tony and I'm in love with two women", except today it was, "Hi, my name is Simon and I've got genital warts." Perhaps telling someone else makes him feel better. Can't say it did the same for me.'

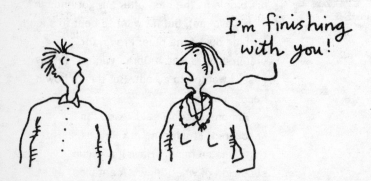

I'm finishing with you!

A SEXUALLY TRANSMITTED
DISEASE – BEING HURT

❛ I've got loads of friends who come up to me and ask if you're supposed to have bumps on your knob. They seem terrified that they've caught something nasty from a toilet seat! ❜

Ben, a medical student from Aberdeen University

Sexually transmitted diseases (STDs)

Sex is great, nice, or at least OK — otherwise forget it. But it can have its down side: getting pregnant when you don't want to, or catching a sexually transmitted disease.

As, on average, people have sex several times a week, and as they also have several sexual partners in a lifetime, there are a lot of STDs being spread around (three-quarters of a million new cases in the UK each year); though given how many people are making love during that time, maybe it isn't all that many.

Most sexually transmitted diseases are caused by bacteria, viruses, yeasts, or the odd spirochaete. However, you are unlikely to catch them except during vaginal intercourse, anal intercourse, or oral sex. Feeling around, touching up, and masturbation are not going to cause a problem.

Some STDs are just a nuisance and are easy to treat. Thrush, for example, which you can get without even having sex and which maybe shouldn't count as an STD. Some keep coming back and are a thorough nuisance, like herpes (remember the joke about 'What is the difference between love and herpes? Herpes lasts forever.'). Some, like chlamydia, can cause future problems like making you infertile. And some, like AIDS, are really BAD NEWS. AIDS cannot be treated and will almost certainly kill you in the end.

Some good things about STDs

◆ if you stick to one partner (and your partner sticks to you!) and you don't start with an STD, you are not likely to get one (except possibly thrush which lurks around)

- you can't catch STDs from toilet seats, doorknobs, or towels

- you can sometimes catch an STD, know you've caught it, and have it treated successfully before it does you any harm, or you pass it on to someone else

- you can cut down the risk of getting an STD by using a condom and/or practising safer sex

- you can get checked out at a genito-urinary clinic (which you can go straight to without a letter)

- you can get checked out by your own GP

Some bad things about STDs

- you can sometimes catch an STD and not know about it

- you can give someone else an STD and not know about it

- some STDs cannot be treated and can continue to give you problems

- some STDs can be treated but will have already caused you damage and may affect your future fertility

- some STDs might lead to cancer in the future

- HIV will almost certainly speed your demise

How not to get an STD

- don't take up sex in the first place

- give up sex now

- don't do it with a stranger

- don't pay for sex

- don't do it with someone who has sores, discharges, or wayward warts

- feel free to have only one STD-free partner

- use a condom

Things may still go wrong, but at least you've tried.

HER

By far the commonest thing you might notice if you have an STD is a change in your vaginal discharge. Almost all women have some discharge, and it is normally non-smelly, slight, and white or clear.

If you have:

- a vaginal discharge which is different from usual (it might be smelly, or more of it, or a different consistency, or a different colour) — **think thrush, trichomonas or bacterial vaginitis** (or if you're very unlucky, all of these). It is less likely to be chlamydia or gonorrhoea

- pain on peeing — **think cystitis — but it could be thrush**

- sores or blisters around the vulva — **think herpes**

- warty lumps around the vagina — **think genital warts**

- itchy/sore vagina — **think thrush**

. . . and then think which one of those clap merchants gave it to me?

HIM

The only two things that normally come out of a man's penis are pee and sperm. However, when you have an STD, other things start coming out, most specifically a discharge (pus, and sometimes blood).

If you have:

- any sort of discharge from the end of your penis — **think gonorrhoea, non-specific urethritis, chlamydia**

- warty lumps on your penis or around it — **think genital warts**

- painful sores or blisters in the same area — **think herpes**

- an itchy willy — **think thrush**

. . . and then think which of the horde gave it to me?

It's worth getting help for any or all of these diseases. You may choose to see your GP (because you could be seeing her for anything); or you may prefer your local genito-urinary medicine (GUM) clinic (because it's more anonymous). If you are really worried that you have an STD, and you want to know immediately, your local GUM clinic is probably the better bet as they can do all the tests and give you the results immediately

There are two other problems which, while they can be associated with sex, do not really count as sexually transmitted diseases as they can occur without being caused by sexual intercourse of any kind. These are cystitis and thrush.

CYSTITIS
This causes pain when you pee, a need to pee more often, desperate feelings of needing to pee immediately, and your pee may look cloudy or red (with blood).

Pauline from London University

The first thing I knew was wetting my knickers while I was trying to get my key in the door. It seemed that as soon as I had finished a pee, I wanted to go again, and the little bit that did come out burnt like hell. All I wanted to do was curl up with a hotty and never drink anything again, so that I wouldn't need to pee.

Cystitis commonly occurs in women, but also occasionally in men, when it is more likely to be due to a sexually transmitted disease — non-specific urethritis. Therefore attacks of cystitis in men should be checked out with a doctor.

It is very common in women and over half the women in this country will suffer from it at some time in their lives — often repeatedly.

It is caused by:

- bacterial germs

- non-bacterial germs (thrush can cause it)

- friction during sex

- allergies (vaginal deodorants, soaps) which all cause inflammation of your urethra and/or bladder

What to do

If you think you've got it, there's a lot you can do to help yourself immediately, and the sooner you start (even in the middle of the night) the sooner it will be over:

- drink a lot (start with a pint of water) to help flush out the germs from the bladder

- if you've got some to hand, add a teaspoonful of bicarbonate of soda (from the chemist or food store and very cheap) to each glass of water. This makes the urine more alkaline which the bugs don't like

- keep drinking

- take some aspirin or paracetamol (whichever suits you)

- keep drinking

- a hot-water bottle covered with a towel on your stomach can be a comfort

- keep drinking (but stay off coffee and alcohol which may make it worse)

If you're still having trouble after a day or two, or if you're getting pain in your back, see a doctor. You may need a short course of antibiotics.

Note: if you keep getting cystitis after you've had sex:

- try washing before and after intercourse (and get your partner to do the same

- pee immediately before and after intercourse

- drink a glass of water with a teaspoonful of bicarbonate of soda in it

- use a lubricant if your vagina is dry, to cut down the friction

If you still feel like doing it after all this, you must be desperate!

THRUSH

This is caused by a type of yeast called *candida albicans* that normally lives on your skin and in your mouth and your gut, minding its own business.

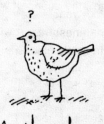

A thrush.

Sarah from Homerton College, Cambridge

❝ I'd been on penicillin (I think that's the reason I got thrush) so I made an emergency appointment. It was a new doctor, and he was very nice and asked me if I wanted a nurse present. I said no, but I felt much less uncomfortable because he asked me that. **The treatment he gave me worked.** ❞

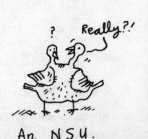

An NSU.

It's a lucky woman who gets through life without ever experiencing thrush. You can get thrush of the mouth, thrush of the vagina, thrush in the gut — and it doesn't have to be caused by sex. If you are taking antibiotics, have diabetes, or are generally unwell, the balance of the normal bugs that hang around in your body all the time gets upset and allows the *candida albicans* yeast to run rampant.

However, sex does play its part (as in everything). Thrush is the most common cause of an itchy vaginal discharge, and can also cause soreness and redness around the vagina, vulva or anus. Sometimes the discharge looks like cottage cheese, which can come as a bit of a surprise. It can be painful to pee or have sex, because the thrush has made everything around the vagina inflamed.

Although sometimes it's only the woman who gets thrush, it can also affect the man's end (so to speak). Men get an itchy, red, sore end to their penis — something of a lighthouse effect — and white spots as well, on occasion.

What to do

There are creams which contain chemicals called fungicides which kill off the yeasts. You can buy these over the counter from any chemist, and Canesten is the most popular. If the soreness is inside the vagina, it's best to buy some special tablets or pessaries to place in the vagina for one to three days until it has all cleared up.

If there's any doubt as to what it is, or if it doesn't clear up after using the cream for a few days, or if you think that the person you were with was a bit dodgy — go and get yourself tested by a doctor. He may send off a swab to the lab to check for bugs under the microscope.

If it keeps coming back, definitely get further advice as there are other treatments available.

You can also help yourself by:

- wearing cotton underwear and avoiding nylon tights and tight trousers

- bathing your vulva in a bath half-full of water with a tablespoon of vinegar in it

- eating live yoghurt (this helps sort out the balance of bugs in your body)

- putting some live yoghurt in your vagina (if you have one)

- dollopping some on to your penis (if you have one)

Yoghurt is a bit messy but it helps for the same reason as eating it helps.

NON-SPECIFIC URETHRITIS (NSU)

This is one of the commonest STDs. NSU is a 'blanket' term for inflammation of the man's urethra (the tube running down the inside of a man's penis). The result is pain — pain in your penis and pain when you pee. You can also get a discharge.

The commonest cause of this inflammation is chlamydia (see below). However, there is no identifiable bug to be found in all people who have NSU, and the bugs that cause it can have been around for some time without causing problems. This means that you could be with a steady partner for some time and suddenly get NSU — either from bugs already in you or from bugs which have been in your partner for some time. Even so, NSU most often happens when you start having sex with a new partner.

Your discharge and your urine need to be tested by a doctor, either at a GUM clinic or by your family doctor. NSU can also be caused by a bug called trichomonas.

What to do

It really is worth getting NSU treated because it can cause infertility. The treatment is a course of antibiotics, and you may need more than one — but antibiotics do work. If your partner/partners don't get treated too, then you are likely to get it again.

CHLAMYDIA

Emily from Durham University

❛ **I think it's scary because you don't always know you've got it.** About three people I know worked out that they all caught it from one person. What was worse was that one girl ended up having to go to hospital because she didn't get treated soon enough.❜

Chlamydia is a common STD, and is caused by a bacteria. It is usually passed on when you have vaginal or anal sex. Sometimes it occurs in people who haven't had a new partner, as the chlamydia bugs can sit around in the body for some time before giving problems; but there's no way you can get it without having had sex.

Women often get infected with chlamydia but don't notice anything. It can cause a vaginal discharge or just extra moisture in the vagina because the chlamydia has inflamed the cells of the cervix making them produce more fluid. In men and women it can also cause inflammation of the urethra making it sting and burn when you pee. In men it sometimes causes a slight, white, cloudy bit of fluid to ooze out from the tip of the penis.

Chlamydia can be a real problem as it can silently damage the Fallopian tubes, causing pelvic inflammatory disease (PID), so it's worth taking care.

Note: With a mild attack of PID the risk of a blocked tube is 3%. With three bad attacks of PID the risk is more like 75%.

What to do

GUM clinics will always test you for chlamydia but your family doctor may not. The GUM clinic is therefore sometimes a better bet. If you go to your family doctor and you're worried about chlamydia, ask for the special test. The treatment is antibiotics, which you may need to take for two weeks.

GENITAL WARTS   *Charlotte from Loughborough University*

❛ **I thought that warts were something you only got on your hands** until I discovered these funny bumps on my vulva. They gave me the fright of my life — but it was the aesthetics of it all that worried me most. *'*

Genital warts are common and are caused by human papilloma viruses. There are thirty different kinds causing verrucas, finger warts, and warts in all sorts of other places. Genital warts, around your penis, vagina, or anus — or even in them (though you may not know you've got them) are usually caught during intercourse.

They may not appear for up to a year after you've caught the virus, though the average time is around three months. Most types of warts don't do much harm, but they certainly aren't very pretty and you may have caught something else at the same time. STDs like company when travelling.

What to do

Depending on where they are, they can be treated, just like hand warts, with a chemical called Podophyllin, which you can get from the doctor. This helps them go, though the virus may still hang about. Some just disappear on their own.

It's the ones you can't see in your partner that you need to worry about, and you can protect against these by using a condom. The ones you can see, you can just say no to.

Warts and the cervix

Women who have certain types of genital wart virus, or have been exposed to these by their partner, are more likely to have an abnormal cervical smear. These changes may indicate a slight increase in the risk of cancer of the cervix in later life. This certainly doesn't mean you're going to get cancer, but it does mean you should have regular smears so that anything abnormal can be treated long before it gets to be a problem.

GENITAL HERPES

Franny from Portsmouth University

' If there is one thing in my life which I really regret and would do something about if I had my time again, it is having caught herpes. I feel totally dirty and furious that he didn't tell me he had herpes himself. I suppose it was because he had only had it once and was probably too embarrassed. I only found out afterwards when I asked him. It wouldn't have stopped me having sex with him, but at least I would have got him to use a condom. Now I've got the bloody thing for a lifetime, and every time I have sex with someone else I've got to tell them.**'**

There are many different kinds of herpes virus. For instance, herpes zoster causes chicken pox, herpes simplex (Type I) causes cold sores, and herpes simplex (Type II) causes genital herpes — but there is a bit of swapping around between these last two.

Some people have just one attack of genital herpes and never have it again, while others get recurrent attacks. You get small clear blisters around the penis or vulva, in the vagina, or around the anus. These blisters burst leaving a painfully sore area. The first attack is always the worst and can make you feel distinctly ill. If you think you might have genital herpes, you shouldn't have sex as the blisters and sores are very infectious to other people. This doesn't mean the end of all sex, but with cold sores — don't kiss, and with genital sores — don't screw or have oral sex. Condoms and Femidoms offer some, but not total, protection.

What is a bit of a problem is that the virus tends to hang around even when you don't have sores. You're unlikely to pass it on then, however. A sign that the blisters are about to come out again is that you get a tingling sensation around your penis or vulva — so you know not to have sex then.

What to do

The good news is that there is a new anti-viral agent called Acyclovir.

This shortens each attack and reduces the number of recurrences, so it's worth taking early. You can get it from your family doctor or a GUM clinic, so don't be embarrassed about getting the diagnosis made.

GONORRHOEA

Yes, it's still around — but not so much of it. It is also known as 'the clap', and is more common among homosexual contacts at the moment. It is only caught by having sex (anal, oral, or vaginal) because it doesn't like living outside the body and needs a nice warm spot like the vagina or urethra. Men know they've got it from about 2 days to 3 weeks after catching it — but beware! Many women don't know they've got it, but can still pass it on. If you have a discharge or soreness, get it checked. The treatment with antibiotics is effective.

What are AIDS and HIV? AIDS stands for 'Acquired Immune Deficiency Syndrome'. It is an infectious disease caused by the Human Immunodeficiency Virus.

Lisa from Oxford University

❛ **I made my boyfriend have an AIDS test because he wouldn't wear a condom or reveal his sexual history to me,** and he'd just been to Sweden. I didn't have a test because it was his choice not to wear a condom. I worried about AIDS when I was entering a long-term relationship, but I've been a bit more careless recently. ❜

Angelo from Leeds University

❛ **It's definitely less romantic,** and something to worry about. It's a niggle at the back of my mind, though a lot of people don't seem to worry at all. If you sleep with a fellow student, you've slept with half the college. ❜

Fiona from Brighton University

❛ **I was worried about whether I'd got glandular fever.** I felt ill and my glands were up. Everyone said I must have got it from kissing, so I went to see my doctor, but what I was really worried about was AIDS.

I felt so stupid. I've always been sensible and used condoms when I've been involved in previous relationships (not that I've had that many). I met this guy when I was on a course, and we went travelling together for a few days. I'd always considered myself really sensible but with this bloke I just got swept off my feet. It must have been his French accent that did it. We had several nights of unbridled — and unprotected — sex.

At first I got really paranoid that I might be pregnant but then my period came OK. But when I became ill with these swollen glands I really started worrying, especially as it was the same day as AIDS Day. Everywhere I looked — newspapers, adverts, the TV — was saying over and over again, "Don't have unprotected sex". I remembered he'd said he had always used condoms in the past, but God did I feel stupid. I wouldn't do it again (at least I hope I wouldn't).

My doctor was reassuring. The chances were small that I had AIDS. But then I started worrying about the AIDS test, partly because of the results and partly because of having to pay more for insurance (and not being able to get life insurance) if I'd had a test. Anyhow, I had it and it was negative. ❜

There is a phenomenon called 'false uniqueness' in student thinking about AIDS. It goes, 'I am somehow different from everyone else and so it won't happen to me, and as everyone else is using precautions, I don't have to.' This represents a kind of 'AIDS invulnerability' — an attitude which is 100 per cent false.

Over a decade since the first case, millions of pounds of research money, millions of cases, and over a million deaths world wide,

and this: **is still the BEST protection.**

A quick facts guide to AIDS and HIV

- the HIV virus is carried in the bloodstream and is transmitted via the blood during sexual intercourse (vaginal or anal), on used needles (and before blood was tested, by blood transfusions). You cannot catch it from kissing, oral sex, touching, lavatory seats, door knobs, drinking glasses, or swimming pools

- on a 'one-off' basis, the chance of catching AIDS during sexual intercourse from an infected partner is between 1 in 100 and 1 in 1,000, with a woman being more likely to catch it from an infected man than vice versa. On the other hand, one-off sexual intercourse is not so common. Would you get in a car if you were told you had a 1 in 100 chance of dying in it during that particular journey?

- you can be tested for the HIV virus but it takes 3 months or more after being infected for the test to go positive

- you are infectious from the moment that you catch it, not from the moment your test is positive

- it can take 10 or more years for someone who is HIV positive to develop symptoms of AIDS, but that person is infectious for all of this time

- most, if not all, infected people will develop AIDS, and die from it or from other illnesses which the HIV virus makes them more susceptible to, such as tuberculosis and some cancers

- most deaths from AIDS in this country at the present time are of homosexuals, intravenous drug users, and haemophiliacs; but the pattern is starting to change. More heterosexuals are now among the new cases and people found to be HIV positive

- if you are about to start a new relationship, are worried you might have caught it, want to sleep with someone who might have caught it (a bisexual, a drug user, a prostitute, a homosexual or a heterosexual who has put him/herself at risk) you can get a test done anonymously by your GP, at a genito-urinary clinic, or at a family planning clinic. You can ask for the results not to be put in your notes and then you needn't worry about insurance companies

- **AIDS cannot yet be cured**

CHAPTER **18**

Feeling lonely, down, out of it, and depressed

Loneliness is ...

- wishing you were someone else

- not having a best friend

- something really bad happening and not being able to tell anyone

- listening to the same music again and again

- waiting around for someone who is always late and wondering whether she will turn up

- people you've never seen before buying you drinks

- being in a strange place, in the pouring rain, for the first time, at 4 p.m. in the afternoon, scrabbling for your front door key, not wanting to go in, opening the door, fumbling for the light switch, collapsing, cold, on your single bed, on your own, with an address book full of people you feel you can't ring

- something inside you feeling as if it's dying

Paul from Durham University

'**Perhaps the reason why many students do not talk about loneliness** is because it is so hard to describe. Sometimes I felt lonely because I had no one to meet for lunch, no one close enough to talk to about my personal problems; sometimes because I had difficulties with my studies, while everyone else seemed to be coping wonderfully. The same type of loneliness never

188

returned twice. It was always a new kind that would suddenly appear, a kind that I never quite knew how to deal with.

Living in a hall of residence surrounded by 170 fellow students who obviously had so much in common made it seem even more ludicrous to feel lonely. But the very reason I felt an outcast was because everyone else seemed to be having such a good time. Now I know differently. When I bring the subject up at the dinner table, people always admit that yes, they did feel lonely at one time or another — we all do.

So why are students unwilling to talk about loneliness — to share the problem? Is it because admitting to feeling lonely is admitting to being a failure? Before university, I was indoctrinated into the belief that we were all going have fun, fun, fun. But university is like a river: **to keep your head above water you have to stay swimming — hard.** 9

Jan from Sussex University

Coping with loneliness

⁶ **I soon realized that feeling lonely is normal** — everyone does. So each time it returned, I did something about it. I phoned my parents, I forced myself to meet some new people by joining societies — even if it involved the sheer terror of going to a first meeting on my own. I learnt to take my mind off my loneliness by concentrating on something else, usually work, which I was good at. I tried not to become obsessed with the idea that people would think me weird for doing things on my own, for instance, walking to lectures by myself, though this was hard.

In reality, I had lots of friends — or enough, at least, but when loneliness did hit me, they suddenly seemed to disappear, or were too preoccupied with their own "good time" to be of any use to me. All I needed was a hug, or a "heart to heart", but even when I don't get those, I know now the misery will pass away. 9

John from Sheffield University

❝ Sometimes I feel that loneliness is like an epidemic waiting to hit the university, full of vulnerable students; yet no one laughs at loneliness, the way they do at exam pressure. They never even bring the topic up. Loneliness seems to be driven inwards. ❞

....

How often do students feel depressed or fed up?   **Depression**

in one study:

▸ **61 in every 100 freshers felt depressed sometimes**

▸ **12 in every 100 felt suicidal at some time**

▸ **4 in every 100 received treatment for depression**

▸ **2 in every 100 suffered from depression every day**

▸ **1 in every 100 had attempted suicide**

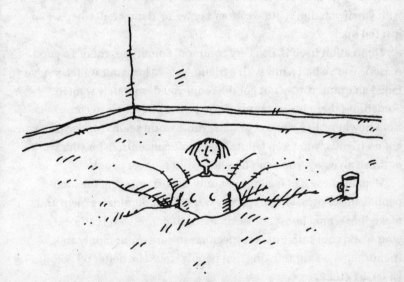

IN A DEPRESSION.

‘ When I got there it was a different story. Shortly after Christmas, I began to get very depressed. I felt fat and ugly next to all the other students, and no blokes ever took an interest in me or my body. I became shy and withdrawn and felt a social outcast. The more withdrawn I became, the more I wanted just to stay in my room, hidden away from everyone. They all intimidated me.

At school I had been very popular and was never short of friends, but suddenly I became hypersensitive to everyone's opinion of me and I would do almost anything to avoid going out with people I didn't know really well. I worried people were talking about me behind my back. I lost the ability to hold a conversation, probably because I was scared of saying something stupid that people would laugh at. Waiting around for tutorials or lectures became a nightmare, watching all those other people talking to one another. **’**

Everyone gets fed up, miserable, and sad. There's something wrong with you if you don't. But we often say we're 'depressed' when we're just fed up.

Depression itself is also very common. Sometimes there's a good reason. You've had a row with a friend, you've lost your wallet, you've failed an exam, you've not got the room you desperately wanted. Sometimes there isn't a reason. Depression just seems to come in from nowhere, like a bad cold. The whole world seems black: you've got no friends, you feel a failure, you can't concentrate on your work or finish an essay, you can't face going out to meet people.

Usually these bad feelings last only a short time. But for some people, the depression can be so severe that it dominates them and makes life seem almost not worth living. If depression is affecting your work, your interests, your feelings towards your family and friends, or you start thinking that people would be better off without you, GET HELP.

Sometimes depression will lift just by talking about it. But if you have more severe symptoms (apathy, lack of concentration, sleep problems, waking early in the morning), then anti-depressant drugs may be very effective. You will not need to go on taking them for ever, and the newer drugs have fewer side-effects than the old ones. It is certainly not a sign of weakness to have to take something.

Where to get help

Parents In most cases, parents will want to help, and will be behind you, whatever happens. Students sometimes forget this, as they don't want to appear as having failed in any way. Put yourself in their position. You'd probably want to know.

Friends They are the best antidote against getting depressed. They can make you laugh and help build up your ego. Most depressed people talk to their friends first, but sometimes you don't want to reveal the cause of a depression to someone you know. One of the advantages of counsellors is that they are not personally involved in your day-to-day affairs.

Your doctor at college Doctors see depression as another illness — like having pneumonia or stomach ache. They will listen to what you have to say, and will try to find out what's worrying you. There are many different ways of dealing with depression. Sometimes talking will be enough, sometimes you will need some tablets, sometimes you will need to see a counsellor or a psychiatrist. Seeing a psychiatrist doesn't mean that you are mad or that this will go on any record — it is all totally confidential. You can tell your doctor what you do or don't want on record, and whether you want him to talk to your tutor or not. It is up to you, but it may sometimes help — especially if you are having trouble with your work.

The college nurse Some colleges and universities employ nurses. They are often trained in counselling students. You may find them very sympathetic and it is worth a try.

The university counselling service Most universities have counselling services. These will be advertised, or you can ask your personal tutor or your doctor. Again, counselling is totally confidential. There is usually an initial session when you talk about your problems, and then you and the counsellor decide together what might help you — perhaps discussing things with the counsellor over a few sessions. It might not seem likely that simply talking about things will help, but most people find that it does.

Susannah from Hertfordshire University

6 It went on for about two weeks. I was sleeping a lot at night, and in the afternoons and evenings. When I was awake, I was either reading, crying, or working. Despite all this, I got good results. It was ridiculous to be feeling like this and I decided I needed help to sort it out.

I went with a friend to the medical centre. I saw a nurse who talked to me for a while and then went off to see someone else. When she came back, she said I could see a counsellor. I was happy about that, I wanted it sorted out.

I started seeing the counsellor once a week. To begin with, I cried more or less for the whole hour, only talking a little; but as the sessions went on, I was gradually crying less and talking more. I don't know how the subjects we discussed came up. The counsellor didn't say much. I liked her a lot. She was kind, she never made judgements, and most of what she said made sense. If it didn't, we tried again. I continued going to see her for two years, until I left college.

It wasn't until I started to feel better that I asked the counsellor what had been wrong. She seemed a little reluctant to tell me, or maybe she was surprised that I hadn't worked it out for myself. Anyway, she said that I had had an identity crisis. The term seemed a bit of a cliché, but the explanation made sense. When I was at home, I had had a definition of myself and what I wanted from life. I was not like my parents, I didn't want to be like them, or live my life the way they did. Although I knew I would have to have a job and earn money, essentially I wanted to have fun and enjoy myself. However, I was defining myself against other things, in a negative way, and when those things were no longer there (like my parents), I was left with nothing to measure myself against, no way to describe myself.

I'm surprised when I look back and realize that I saw the counsellor for so long. It didn't seem like that at the time. I remember when the sessions were drawing to an end, I didn't want them to stop — to be left to manage on my own. **9**

Negative thoughts can be infectious, and seem to feed on each other in one's mind. Something like this:

Negative thought blocking

6 I've got nothing to wear, well, nothing that really suits me. That's because I'm not very attractive, so no one is going to like me. I have no friends, have I? So what's the point of going to this party, anyway? But if I don't go, there's nothing else to do — but sit around and be miserable. **9**

The art is to stop this train of thought as early as possible. As soon as you realize you are off down this negative track, start blocking the thoughts with positive thoughts instead. Say to yourself, 'Hey, hold on, what's all this about? What do I need this hassle for? Is it going to serve any useful purpose? Why don't I block it with some really positive thoughts instead?'

6 I bet my girlfriend is going to go off with someone else.
But I do have quite a few admirers who could step into her shoes, and anyway she actually does seem to like me a lot. We have gone out four times in the last week, and I don't know that she's off with someone else. **9**

❛ I'm behind with my work.
But I'm conscientious and have always managed to catch up before. There's no reason for it to be any different now, and my tutor said my last essay was terrific. ❜

❛ I always feel shy about talking to people.
But I'm good with words and can actually make people laugh, if I can remember the jokes. Last time I got smashed out of my mind, people could hardly get me to stop talking. And anyway, it's not "always" — just occasionally. ❜

❛ Spots again, and everyone said they'd stop when I stopped being a teenager.
Well actually, you can hardly see them and I've got a tube of Clearasil. It hasn't stopped my girlfriend yet, and John's got much worse spots than me. ❜

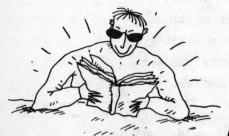

A 'bright thoughts' diary

**Monday
20th December**

There are a few things I'm interested in and think I'd like to do.

I am enjoying some of my work, for the first time for ages.

I can be quite witty (when not entirely neurotic).

Sometimes I feel despairing because some worries insist on returning. What shall I do next term? Will I spend enough time with other people? And what do I want to do with my life?

Tuesday **21st December**	My birthday. Feel awful, as I'm supposed to be enjoying myself.

Thursday **23rd December**	I am quite creative.
	I'm good at using words.
	I have managed to get my parents' Christmas presents.
	I am not totally devoid of opinions, and managed to tell a friend that what he thought was good was actually trash.

Friday **24th December**	I do have a number of friends.
	I am conscientious.
	I fit into most groups — except that all too elusive football crowd at uni.
	I managed a game of pool at the pub today.

Saturday **25th December**	I got a number of presents from people I thought had forgotten me.
	I did not depart immediately after dinner, and was not the first to go.
	I made two jokes which people laughed at.

Sunday **26th December**	I've got properly involved in a book (quite an achievement for me).
	I am interested in acquiring self-confidence.
	I'm concerned about people less fortunate than myself.
	I can see depression could be a useful experience.

CHAPTER 19

To eat or not to eat? That is the question

The experiences of others

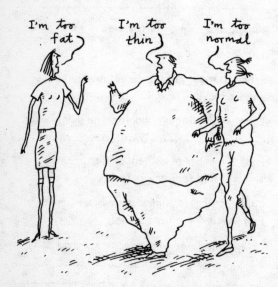

Jane from Manchester University

'I met many students who were also suffering from eating disorders and anorexia. This illness seems to be largely derived from the same reserve, self-discipline, perseverance, and iron will that got us into university in the first place.'

Anthea from East London University

'On entering university I felt a desperate need to fit in. I carried with me this guilty secret of having been sexually abused as a child. However, what actually happened was that I became a social recluse as a result of ignoring everyone around me, and I developed this eating disorder known as bulimia. For a while, the issue of food had paramount importance and dominated my studies, my relationships, and, above all, me. I constantly worried about how fat I was and whether I was doing enough exercise, forgetting about my dwindling finances in my efforts to buy laxatives and food for the constant binges which occupied my life. Eventually those around me began to notice, but this made me feel even more alienated and lonely, and I withdrew further into myself. I found it incredibly difficult to ask for help.'

When eating it is <u>OK</u> to:

- enjoy it
- eat some junk foods without feeling guilty
- eat at least three times a day
- vary the amount you eat from day to day
- eat more of what you like and less of what you don't like
- eat a variety of different foods
- eat enough food not to feel hungry all the time
- eat with other people

When eating it is <u>not</u> OK to:

- always be on a diet
- count the calorie value of every scrap of food
- be obsessed about your weight
- eat so little that you always feel hungry
- treat any foods as absolutely forbidden
- weigh yourself every day

Eating habits   Our eating habits vary enormously. Some of us appear to eat huge amounts of food and manage to stay thin, others appear to eat little and get fat. Some eat three regular meals a day, others 'snack' throughout the day — in much the same way as some of us are tall and some short, and some have fair hair, some dark.

It is difficult to know when 'normal' eating merges into 'abnormal' eating; but it has gradually become obvious that eating disorders are more common nowadays than they used to be, are more common in 'developed' societies, and more common among young people of student age.

How much should you weigh?

Your weight varies from day to day because of what food is inside
your guts and also the amount of fluid washing around you at any one
time. A variation of up to 3lb (over a kilo) is quite normal. This
completely negates the value of daily weighing. Weekly weighing on
the same scales, at the same time of day, is the maximum
recommended frequency, and if you really want to judge whether your
weight is going up or down, monthly intervals are the most useful.

What is usually measured nowadays is the 'Body Mass Index' or
BMI. This is your weight in kilograms divided by the square of your
height in metres. There is no absolute 'right' for your BMI, but it
should be greater than 18. The average is 20 to 25, and if it's more
than 30, you are overweight.

Eating disorders

There are two main types of eating
disorder, and over-concern about body
shape and weight are common to both.

Anorexia nervosa, which is common among teenagers, basically
results in people being very controlled about what they eat and
becoming very thin.

Bulimia nervosa is when people of normal weight or who are
overweight go in for dieting, followed by binge eating and then self-
induced vomiting. This is common among young adults.

There is some overlap between the two disorders, and one can
lead to the other. Only about 1 in 10 people with eating disorders
seeks help. This is because many feel guilty about it, which is a pity
as, contrary to popular myth, there is a lot that can be done to help.
Most of these remedies are simple and don't involve seeing a
psychiatrist or going into hospital.

We are not sure why girls are more likely to suffer from eating
disorders than boys. The influences of media pressure may well play
a part. You have only to look at women's magazines where 'slim
is beautiful'.

Why are students vulnerable to eating disorders?

Some factors that may contribute:

- moving into a college environment and losing the security of family and familiar friends who accept you as you are

- getting established in a new social scene which makes you feel vulnerable, both emotionally and physically; you become self-conscious about the way you look and behave

- having to feed yourself, at odd times of day, with no fixed meal times

- more privacy in which to binge and make yourself vomit at will

Anorexia nervosa This is when you deliberately choose to lose weight to such an extent that you are 15% (or more) below the expected minimum that is normal for your height. This is what separates anorexia nervosa from ordinary slimming. Not everyone who is slim is anorexic!

Anorexia is not just a question of not eating, but also of using laxatives and taking excessive exercise — like running five miles a day.

Nobody knows why it happens, though there are various theories, which include: wanting to put off the demands of maturing, especially sexual demands; wanting to stay a child; wanting to gain attention within the family.

Although the problem is in the mind (body image and suchlike), most of the results are purely physical. People with anorexia begin to look very thin — though they think of themselves as overweight and fat. They become irritable and humourless. Concentration goes, tiredness creeps in, work suffers. These symptoms are all the result of lack of food: starvation. When sufferers start eating again, they all disappear.

Because anorexics are so thin, they are sensitive to the cold and their hands and feet turn blue or red when the temperature goes down. Their hormones get all upset, women stop having periods and get more hairy, and both men and women lose interest in sex (which may be a relief for some).

One characteristic of anorexics is that they think they are getting more and more attractive, while it is perfectly obvious to everyone around that they are actually looking increasingly ghastly. At the same time, they are totally denying that anything is wrong or that they have any kind of eating problem.

What to do

If this applies to you, admit you've got a problem and get some help. If it applies to your friend, get that friend to admit the problem (which may be difficult) and point her or him towards a GP, university counsellor, nurse, tutor, or the national self-help anorexic group called Anorexic Aid.

Some people find that reading about others' experiences can be a great help and makes them feel less isolated. Try reading:
Women's Secret Disorder, by Mira Dana and Marilyn Lawrence (Grafton Books, 1988).
When Food Is Love, by Geneen Roth (Piatkus, 1992).
Eating Disorders: The Facts, by Susan Abraham and Derek Llewellyn Jones (Oxford University Press, 1992).

Simple self-help measures

- **stop counting calories (or for at least one meal a day)**
- **stop weighing food (or for at least one meal a day)**
- **try eating with other people**

....

Jody from Manchester University

⁶Bulimia is a horrific, time-consuming, and degrading business. It **Bulimia** is a shield, it is a sword, it is a method of torture that many women and some men put themselves through every hour, every day, every week, every month. To my horror, bulimia has sometimes been labelled "the fashionable illness" — suffering for the sake of a flat stomach, thin thighs, and a tiny frame, all in order to conform to society's ideal of a "perfect body". Instead it is an outlet for despair, hopelessness, unhappiness, guilt, shame and anger . . . the list goes on. It is something I went through, and survived.

Food has always been my best friend and my worst enemy. As a child, I loved food with a voracious appetite, but hated my body. I detested going swimming or holidaying because bikinis were a nightmare. I couldn't even face myself in the mirror, let alone let anyone else see me. I felt uncomfortable walking around in my own flesh.

As I grew up into adolescence the problem increased. Developing breasts and "a figure" was frightening: I felt my sexuality was staring people in the face. I hated the aura that my body projected, and I was scared of physical contact with boys — their wandering hands, their endless curiosity. My body was mine and no one else's. My mother despaired, and even questioned me on my sexual orientation, though all I wanted to be was sexless. In all this, food began to play a greater and greater role.

At university, the freedom to hoard food and shut the door to the outside world, allowed me to relieve myself of my anxieties by huge binges of secret eating: biscuits, cakes, crisps, baked beans, cheese, tinned meat, loaves of bread . . . binge, binge, binge — then a vomiting session. I would clean myself up, open the door, and try and present the perfect woman to the outside world.

If my day didn't go as planned, if I was stressed on an essay, if someone said something I didn't like — off I went to eat. I just couldn't weather emotion, and bingeing and vomiting gave me the control I was looking for. While all else in my life fell apart, at least I was in charge of what I ate.

My weight ballooned, my face puffed up, my gums grew sore, my vocal cords became raw. I became paranoid about my size, subjected myself to bouts of starvation, my moods swung backwards and forwards, and I became a walking disaster. No one noticed. After all, I put my other mask on when I went out. All I wanted was to be thin. If I was thin, I would be beautiful. If I was beautiful, I would feel strong, with no problems.

Being a perfectionist in my work and in everything else I did, I wanted "perfection" in my looks. In this age of glossy magazines, glamorous soap operas, and fascination with sex, we are continually subjected to pictures telling us what we should look like. They encapsulate the view that thinness and beauty are the keys to success, happiness, and loving relationships. I never felt loved for who I was, but for what I was expected to be.

Talking about all this to my GP, admitting it, crying, shouting, expressing my pent-up anger, and telling others how I really am, helped me to break out of the rut. With the help of my GP at university, I learned how to follow a proper diet, respect my bodily needs, and understand food as a normal, vital element for living. I worked through my depression, learnt how to be good to myself, to look in the mirror and see reality. It's not easy, and I still wake each morning hoping that my stomach is flatter and my thighs thinner, but I can now look in the mirror and like what I see.

The thing is to understand what is happening, to admit and accept that you need help, and to seek it actively.[9]

The binger and the binges

Binge eating is the main symptom of bulimia, usually followed by a feeling of lack of control over the whole business (whereas anorexics feel they have total control). Bulimics then induce vomiting, use laxatives, and take excessive exercise, followed by some strict dieting and fasting, followed in turn by some more binge eating. To 'join the club' (fulfil the American criteria put out by the American Psychiatric Association) you have to binge eat at least twice a week for three months or more.

Bingers are usually ashamed of their behaviour and are secretive about it all. During a bingeing day, the binger can eat up to thirty times what a normal individual would consume over the same period

— 20,000 kcal plus. Some will deliberately binge on fatty foods which they normally wouldn't touch. The food is often eaten rapidly in great gulps, and if you have these excessive binges, you are likely to be overweight — even if you try and vomit afterwards.

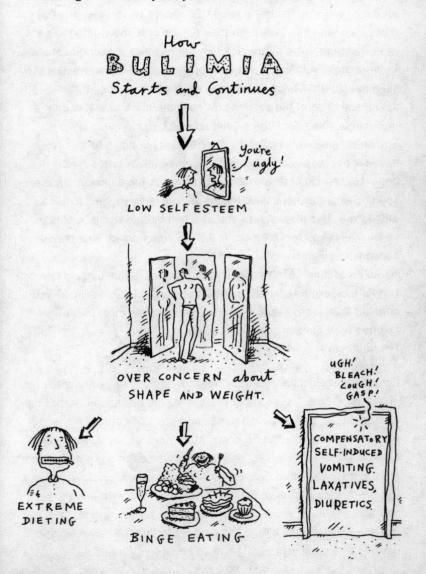

After a binge, the binger feels guilty and depressed, and vows to go on a strict diet, even to starve for a long period — until the next binge (which may be up to twenty times a day, or two or three times a week).

Sometimes the drive to overeat goes on for weeks at a time, and six out of every ten bulimics force themselves to vomit on a regular basis. To start with, they push their fingers or a spoon into the back of their throat, but with practice they can manage it spontaneously. Unfortunately, vomiting is not a particularly good way of avoiding the calories. Most bulimics do not lose weight as they absorb the calories in spite of the vomiting. At absolute maximum, it is only possible to vomit back three-quarters of a binge.

The downside of regular vomiting is that you begin to look like a hamster because your salivary glands swell up. Your teeth rot because the acid from your stomach removes the enamel from them. The chemical balances in your body get upset so you feel exhausted and unwell. This also causes you to retain more water in your body, which makes you feel bloated; and if you're a woman, your periods become irregular.

As if vomiting wasn't enough after bingeing, some bingers take handfuls of laxatives, which can be dangerous. They may make you crap but this doesn't reduce your weight because most of the calories have already been absorbed in the gut.

What to do

People with bulimia desperately want to eat normally, without the fear of gaining weight. The secret of overcoming the disorder is, surprisingly, to stop dieting and establish a regular pattern of eating. This is because people who diet have very strict rules about calorie intake, allowable foods, and eating only at certain times of day. Anyone who tries to stick to such a rigid set of rules is doomed to failure. When you break the rules, even in little ways, which is inevitable, you feel bad about yourself and totally out of control, so you give up for the day and binge, binge, binge. The paradox is that the very rules you develop to control your eating end up being your downfall.

A DAY'S EATING DIARY

Time	Food & Drink	Place	Excessive (Y/N)?	V/L?	Comments
8.30am	Orange juice Black coffee	Room	No		It's going to be a good day
2.30pm	Cheese sandwich 1 doughnut	Outside library	Y/N		
2.35pm	Mars Bar 1 doughnut (only ate half of this)	In library	Yes		Starving, can't stop myself Will not eat much for supper
8.10pm	Toast Cottage cheese 1 tomato 1 diet Lilt	Communal kitchen	No		Missed hall-food. Too stodgy No good vegetarian
9.00pm	1 large kettle crisps	Room	Yes!		
9.10pm	Bowl of cereal 2 cups of tea More toast	Room	Yes	V	Weighed myself – 9st 3lbs – cried
10.00pm	Crisps, nuts 1 pint of beer	Bar	Yes	V	Felt bloated Can't go on Just hate myself

V/L = Vomiting or laxatives

Self-help

- keep a diary of what you are eating

- try to have two or three planned meals a day, plus one or two planned snacks

- try not to work in your room where you can binge eat at liberty; work in public places like libraries instead

- don't go more than three hours without eating

- don't weigh yourself more than once a week

- if you stop bingeing you are very unlikely to gain weight because overall you are not eating so much

- write down a list of alternative action for when you want to binge: phoning a friend, buying a book, having a bath, going for a walk

- arrange to have all your meals with friends

- avoid situations which you know result in binge eating

- limit the amount of food available to you when eating

- practise leaving some food on the plate

- throw away any leftover foods

- stay away from your binge foods to begin with

- shop with a shopping list drawn up when you are not hungry

- always sit down to eat

- contact your Women's Officer, who will put you in touch with local support groups

> There is a book you might like to read about bulimia
>
> *Bulimia Nervosa: A Guide to Recovery,* by Peter J. Cooper (Robinson Health, 1993).

Helping a friend

If a friend with an eating disorder comes to you for help, try to find out as much as you can about the problem (like reading this chapter, and maybe other books — see above). Ask your friend to tell you about it, and try to persuade her to get some help from her family doctor or a student counsellor. You, as a student yourself, cannot take on the therapeutic role, and you should not collude in any secrecy.

If you suspect a friend has an eating disorder but won't admit it, let her know that you know, as that might get her to confront the problem. You can show her this chapter and see if it helps. You mustn't collude with her, and you mustn't take on the guilt for her problems. You can, however, offer friendship and support.

Suicidal *Feelings*

Suicidal thoughts? You're not alone ... All students sometimes get to feel that life is a bitch, and some feel that they don't want to go on living. But these feelings usually pass, some distraction happens, or another, more positive bit of thinking comes to mind. At least 10 per cent of students have, at one time or another during their student days, felt suicidal, and up to 3 per cent have attempted suicide.

It doesn't mean you're mad, bad or peculiar if you do have suicidal thoughts. You can feel totally black one moment and much better a few hours later. There's a whole range of untimely intrusions, from vague thoughts of death through to hard core determination. There's also a range of things which people actually try, from mild attempts at self-harm (which can be a cry for help) through to the very rare moment when someone plans to kill himself with care and forethought, and it happens.

❝ Well, I suppose we all feel suicidal from time to time, but it's hardly the thing I tell everyone. ❞ Now that I have told a few people, it appears that everyone in the whole world has the same feelings. I'm not sure whether knowing I'm not alone in occasionally feeling totally miserable makes it better — or worse. Part of the suicidal feeling is being sorry for myself, and now it turns out I've got to feel sorry for everyone else too. It doesn't happen all that often, just often enough to start wondering what the best way of doing it would be . . . ❞

❝ On Wednesday morning, after the party, I went home and took three sleepers and as much whisky as I could ❞ — just because I had no dope and wanted to become high. I also wrote a suicide note, but I couldn't bring myself to do it, so I ended up both pissed and drowsy. Isabel came over and stayed the night, and we talked, cried and made love.

Thursday was OK, but on Thursday night I went out with John and his friends. Once again, his way of trying to help me deal with it all was to say, "Come out with us, take some speed, and you'll feel great." I didn't, but the next day I was so upset, and on my own in the hall of residence, that once again I took some sleepers (five this time) and some gin — and then I phoned the Samaritans. They listened, and made me open up to the fact that I needed help.

Then I did another good thing, considering the state I was in. I phoned my doctor and after fifteen minutes he came round. He called my mum, because I asked him to. And then I decided that as I was afraid of myself at that moment, I wanted to go to a safe place. That evening I went into the local psychiatric hospital and was admitted over the weekend. ❞

❝ When I heard that Mat had committed suicide, I thought "Oh no, if only I had..." ❞ I guess it was just me feeling guilty — but I did feel guilty. I knew he was down. We all get down. It was ridiculous, he would have got a first even if he hadn't done any work between now and the exam. And you can't really blame

Tammy for leaving him — it just wasn't working.
He'd seemed OK when I saw him on the
Saturday. I'd meant to meet him on the Sunday,
but somehow I didn't get around to it. **I just
can't believe I won't see him again.**⁹

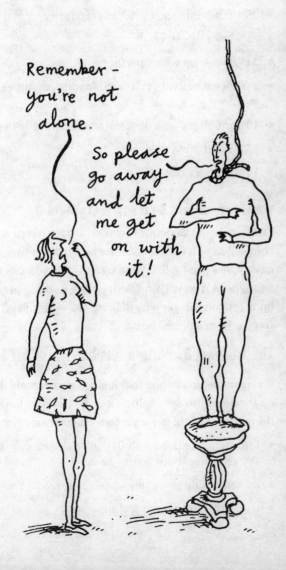

From one study, the most common problems cited by students who have attempted suicide (often several reasons are given) are as follows:

- 33% difficulty with their studies

- 31% problems with their parents

- 26% academic and career uncertainties

- 25% low self-esteem

- 24% break-up with a partner

- 24% problems with relationships with their peers (but not with partners)

- 19% problems with ongoing relationships with partners

- 15% exam pressures

- 14% feeling isolated

What you should do if you feel suicidal

You should tell someone — a friend, your parents, a tutor, a counsellor, or a GP (who should be available twenty-four hours a day). If you can't tell anyone face to face, you can always ring the Samaritans. You will find their phone number in the local phone book (or you can get it by dialling 192 — which is free if you're ringing from a phone box).

The national Samaritan number is: 071-734 2800

If you are feeling depressed, it is often extremely difficult to summon up the energy to seek help. It may be that you have to do some little thing to start with, to get underway, such as:

- find someone to be with (if you're alone), even if you don't want to say anything about feeling suicidal

- do something you enjoy — exercise, read a book

- try writing down your feelings

- try asking yourself what you need this depression for
- climb into bed and try to sleep

If there is nothing that the depression is useful for, try mentally discarding it. This can take a bit of practice!

What you should do if friends feel suicidal

- try to get them to talk to you about how they are feeling
- if they say they would be better off dead, take it seriously and get them some help
- encourage them to discuss how they feel with someone else, their tutor, their doctor, counsellor or nurse; the Samaritans or a student help-line

While it is important not to go around blabbing what a fellow student has told you in confidence, mention of suicide is usually an exception to this rule. You should talk to one of the tutors or lecturers; if possible, someone who knows the student concerned. This may seem rather deceitful to your friend, but it may also be effective in stopping him or her from committing suicide.

> **It is not true that people who talk about suicide don't do it — _they do._**

Some facts and figures

More men than women actually succeed in killing themselves. In the student population, the ratio is roughly three times as many men as women. Suicide is increasing among young men. It is now the second most common cause of death.

Since 1980, **actual** suicides of young men have risen dramatically — an 85% increase among 16 to 24-year-olds. Why is this? We don't really know, though some or all of the following may play a part:

- increasing rates of unemployment
- increasing use of alcohol

- drug taking
- family breakdown
- AIDS
- influence of the media (including saying how other students have done it)
- psychiatric problems

The number of **actual** suicides among young women has fallen slightly, though the rates of attempted suicide are higher in young women than in men. The rates have remained stable for the last few years.

Among young people in general who attempt suicide, the most frequently given reasons are problems with relationships. Unemployment and alcohol and drug problems are also common — especially among men.

The last word

When all is said and done, the ultimate goal of it all ...

❝ *But honestly, any worries I have are overridden by the complete joy of actually having managed it. I know that some of my friends, who didn't make it, will absolutely hate me for saying that. But it is the excitement of starting a completely new life, with a whole set of new experiences, and doing something that I really wanted to do. I'm sure there will be ups and downs — that's what life's about, isn't it, taking the rough with the smooth? You've just got to try and get the most out of it, whatever happens.* **❞**

AFTER –

Why on earth can't I be a student all my life?

INDEX